Foundations in

Patient Safety for
Health Professionals

Edited by

Kimberly A. Galt, RPh, PharmD, FASHP

Professor and Associate Dean for Research
Director
Creighton Center for Health Services Research and Patient Safety
Creighton University

Karen A. Paschal, PT, DPT, MS

Associate Professor
Department of Physical Therapy
Creighton Center for Health Services Research and Patient Safety
Creighton University

JONES AND BARTLETT PUBLISHERS
Sudbury, Massachusetts
BOSTON   TORONTO   LONDON   SINGAPORE

World Headquarters

Jones and Bartlett Publishers
40 Tall Pine Drive
Sudbury, MA 01776
978-443-5000
info@jbpub.com
www.jbpub.com

Jones and Bartlett Publishers
Canada
6339 Ormindale Way
Mississauga, Ontario L5V 1J2
Canada

Jones and Bartlett Publishers
International
Barb House, Barb Mews
London W6 7PA
United Kingdom

Jones and Bartlett's books and products are available through most bookstores and online booksellers. To contact Jones and Bartlett Publishers directly, call 800-832-0034, fax 978-443-8000, or visit our website, www.jbpub.com.

Substantial discounts on bulk quantities of Jones and Bartlett's publications are available to corporations, professional associations, and other qualified organizations. For details and specific discount information, contact the special sales department at Jones and Bartlett via the above contact information or send an email to specialsales@jbpub.com.

This publication is designed to provide accurate and authoritative information in regard to the Subject Matter covered. It is sold with the understanding that the publisher is not engaged in rendering legal, accounting, or other professional service. If legal advice or other expert assistance is required, the service of a competent professional person should be sought.

Production Credits

Publisher: David Cella
Acquisitions Editor: Kristine Jones
Associate Editor: Maro Gartside
Editorial Assistant: Teresa Reilly
Production Director: Amy Rose
Senior Production Editor: Renée Sekerak
Marketing Manager: Grace Richards
Manufacturing and Inventory Control
  Supervisor: Amy Bacus

Cover and Title Page Design: Kate Ternullo
Cover Images: Pharmacist © Diego Cervo/
  ShutterStock, Inc.; Doctor with patient and
  nurse with patient © Monkey Business
  Images/ShutterStock, Inc.; Background
  © kentoh/ShutterStock, Inc.
Composition: Glyph International
Printing and Binding: Malloy Incorporated
Cover Printing: Malloy Incorporated

Library of Congress Cataloging-in-Publication Data
Galt, Kimberly A.
  Foundations in patient safety for health professionals/Kimberly A. Galt, Karen A. Paschal.
     p. ; cm.
  Includes bibliographical references and index.
  ISBN 978-0-7637-6338-1 (alk. paper)
  1. Hospitals—Safety measures. 2. Medical
errors—Prevention. 3. Medication errors—Prevention. I. Paschal, Karen A. II. Title.
  [DNLM: 1. Medical Errors—prevention & control—United States. 2. Patient Care
—methods—United States. 3. Risk Assessment—United States. 4. Safety Management
—methods—United States. WB 100 G179f 2010]
  RA969.9.G35 2010
  362.11068'4—dc22

                                                                    2009035642

6048

Printed in the United States of America
13 12 11 10 09   10 9 8 7 6 5 4 3 2 1

This book is dedicated to

Mike,
Ryan, Christine, and Jenee
and Sandy

Pat,
Becky, Juande, and Lucía,
Katie and Neel

May the lessons learned by those who read this book help to
make your health care safer.

Contents

Foreword

The 1999 release of the Institute of Medicine (IOM) report, *To Err Is Human*,[1] was a wake-up call for American health professionals and institutions. It created great concern and a heightened awareness that all is not well in American health care, and it sparked a national effort to address the human and system flaws that result in medical errors. The subsequent release of the second report of the IOM Committee on Quality of Health Care in America, *Crossing the Quality Chasm*,[2] laid out strategies for addressing and reducing errors, including system and institutional design change, development, and application of evidence to the study of errors, aligning payment with quality, and enhancing the education of health professionals.

In 2002, the IOM convened a Health Professions Education Summit that produced a third report, *Health Professions Education: A Bridge to Quality*.[3] This report defined five core competencies of health professionals necessary to improve quality, reduce errors, and assure patient safety. Competent health professionals should provide patient-centered care, work in interdisciplinary teams, employ evidence-based practice, apply quality improvement, and utilize informatics.

In 2003, in response to the clear need to address the development of students' competence to work in interdisciplinary teams, Creighton University established an Office of Interprofessional Education, of which I was named director. Several interprofessional teams were assembled to plan and implement educational experiences to offer students of Creighton's health professions schools and programs. One of the interprofessional teams, comprising expertise in law, medicine, nursing, pharmacy, physical therapy, occupational therapy, social work, systems design, and decision sciences, embarked on the development of an interprofessional course in Patient Safety offered to students in several colleges and schools within the university. It is that course and the experiences of its faculty who are teaching that have given rise to this book.

As pioneers, course faculty quickly found that there was no extant text available that met the needs of their students. In consequence, they embarked on distilling the essence of the course to develop the present comprehensive text and approach to teaching patient safety to a group of students drawn from a variety of professions. This is an interprofessional faculty teaching an interprofessional student body.

This text presents the background and need for safety improvement, why errors occur, principles of patient safety assurance, quality and safety improvement, the appropriate and constructive use of evidence, the importance of systems design, and organizational structure and culture. It also addresses questions of safety from patients' and professionals' perspectives and, very importantly, the responsibilities of professionals, employers, and organizations when errors occur, when patient safety is compromised, or when patients are injured.

The work will be of great value to similar interprofessional teams teaching students drawn from a variety of professional backgrounds, including not only the health professions but also management, law, systems design, decision sciences, and information technology.

Richard L. O'Brien

Richard L. O'Brien, MD, FACP

Richard O'Brien is University Professor and a member of the Center for Health Policy and Ethics at Creighton University. He was a participant in the 2002 Institute of Medicine Health Professions Education Summit and in 2003 was appointed director of the Office of Interprofessional Education at Creighton, a position he held until 2006. During his tenure in this office he instigated and assisted the development of a number of interprofessional education activities for students of business, law, dentistry, medicine, nursing, occupational therapy, pharmacy, physical therapy, and social work. He was also dean of the School of Medicine at Creighton from 1982 to 1992 and vice president for Health Sciences from 1984 to 1999. He and two colleagues have recently published a book, *Cultural Proficiency in Addressing Health Disparities* (also published by Jones and Bartlett). He is currently engaged in studying and teaching the ethics of health policy formation, human subject research, and the reduction of health disparities.

REFERENCES

1. Committee on Quality of Health Care in America, Institute of Medicine, Kohn LT, Corrigan JM, Donaldson MS (eds). *To Err Is Human—Building a Safer Health System*, National Academy Press, Washington, DC, 2000.
2. Committee on Quality of Health Care in America, Institute of Medicine, *Crossing the Quality Chasm: A New Health System for the 21st Century*, National Academy Press, Washington, DC, 2001.
3. Committee on Health Professions Education Summit, Board on Health Care Services, Institute of Medicine, Greine AC, Knebel E (eds). *Health Professions Education: A Bridge to Quality*, National Academy Press, Washington, DC, 2003.

Acknowledgments

Why would 15 faculty members from across a university campus, with no particular reason to work together, establish solidarity in our commitment to teaching students about the sciences of patient safety?

There is only one reason. Each of us has a personal story. The story is one of harm and injury through errors, mishaps, and mistakes. For some of us the story describes the pain, suffering, or losses of our own loved ones. For others, the story illustrates the pain, suffering, or losses incurred by others we tried to care for through our own professional experiences.

And while each story is unique to the persons or places involved, all stories share a common and powerful feature—isolation. Each of us had not discussed our own personal story with others to any great extent. Where would one go to do that? Where is the support system or vehicle for communication with each other about this? Let's face it; we had an unusual and rare experience, didn't we? What happened couldn't possibly be frequently encountered by others, we rationalized.

But our experiences are frequently encountered by others. The overwhelming body of evidence has repetitively shown us this truth. And even more astounding is that we know that much of this harm and injury is avoidable. Avoidable if we each take responsibility for being competent at and applying safety principles to patient care delivery.

We are indebted to those who have brought this most important area of care and concern into the visible forefront of our social priorities—the scientists, clinicians, and advocates for patient safety. Most of all, we are grateful to the individuals and families who have experienced harm, but are willing to share their stories with the hope of making a difference in the lives of others.

Contributors

Amy A. Abbott, PhD, RN

Amy Abbott is an assistant professor and faculty member in the School of Nursing at Creighton University and in the Creighton Center for Health Services Research and Patient Safety, as well as a staff nurse at Creighton University Medical Center in the Adult Intensive Care Unit. Dr. Abbott's research interests include patient safety and quality in nursing education and practice and health information technology. She has been actively involved in the multidisciplinary patient safety course since 2007. Dr. Abbott is a Patient Safety Expert Panel Reviewer for the Creighton Center for Health Services Research and Patient Safety, Patient Safety Organization.

James D. Bramble, PhD, MPH

James D. Bramble is an associate professor in the School of Pharmacy and Health Professions and the Director of the Health Services Administration Certificate Program at Creighton University. Dr. Bramble teaches courses on research methodology and biostatistics, as well as healthcare management and patient safety. His research focuses on patient safety, health information technology, and resource utilization in healthcare organizations. He has been involved in many funded grant projects, published in both books and health science research journals, had book reviews accepted for publication, been an adjunct journal reviewer, and has presented at many conferences and meetings. Dr. Bramble also has a secondary appointment in the School of Medicine's Department of Anesthesiology and has held a Creighton Center for Health Services Research and Patient Safety faculty membership since 2004. He participates in the interprofessional education course Foundations in Patient Safety. Dr. Bramble is a Patient Safety Expert Panel Reviewer for the Creighton Center for Health Services Research and Patient Safety, Patient Safety Organization.

Bartholomew E. Clark, RPh, PhD

Bartholomew E. Clark is an associate professor in the School of Pharmacy and Health Professions at Creighton University. Before earning a PhD in the Social and Administrative Sciences in Pharmacy at the University of Wisconsin–Madison, Dr. Clark earned a BS in Pharmacy and an MS in Pharmacy Administration at the University of Illinois at Chicago, practiced pharmacy in a variety of community and institutional settings, and served as Professional Affairs Manager at the National Association of Boards of Pharmacy. Dr. Clark's research interests include patient safety and professional and workplace attributes that contribute to pharmacists' organizational commitment. Responsibilities at Creighton include teaching in Pharmacy Practice Management, Pharmacy Practice Law, and Foundations in Patient Safety. Dr. Clark is a Patient Safety Expert Panel Reviewer for the Creighton Center for Health Services Research and Patient Safety, Patient Safety Organization.

Teresa M. Cochran, PT, DPT, GCS, MA

Teresa M. Cochran is an associate professor and vice chair in the Department of Physical Therapy, School of Pharmacy and Health Professions, Creighton University, Omaha, Nebraska. She also codirects the Office of Interprofessional Scholarship, Service, and Education and is a faculty affiliate in the Center for Health Policy and Ethics at Creighton University. Dr. Cochran's teaching responsibilities are focused in the areas of behavioral science and evidence-based decision making in the entry-level and transitional Doctor of Physical Therapy programs. She earned specialist board certification in geriatric physical therapy from the American Board of Physical Therapy Specialties, and her research interests explore practice errors in rehabilitation, access to rehabilitation for vulnerable groups, and prevention of chronic conditions and disability. Dr. Cochran currently serves as president of the Nebraska Chapter of the American Physical Therapy Association. Dr. Cochran is a Patient Safety Expert Panel Reviewer for the Creighton Center for Health Services Research and Patient Safety, Patient Safety Organization.

Andjela Drincic, MD

Andjela Drincic is a faculty member at the Creighton Center for Health Services Research and Patient Safety (CHRP) and associate professor of Medicine at Creighton University School of Medicine. As a member of CHRP, she has been involved in research focusing on error identification and prevention in both inpatient and outpatient settings. As a medical director for diabetes services at Creighton University Medical Center, she is working on prevention of insulin errors in the hospital environment. She has specific interest in human-technology safety issues in the outpatient endocrinology clinics. She, along with the coauthors of this book, has been teaching the campus-wide interdisciplinary patient safety course since 2005. Dr. Drincic is a Patient Safety Expert Panel Reviewer for the Creighton Center for Health Services Research and Patient Safety, Patient Safety Organization.

Kevin T. Fuji, PharmD

Kevin Fuji is an Assistant Professor and also recently completed his program as a Health Services Research Fellow with an emphasis in Patient Safety for the Creighton Center for Health Services Research and Patient Safety in the School of Pharmacy and Health Professions at Creighton University. He conducts research examining the adoption and use of health information technologies, specifically personal and electronic health records, in the context of patient safety and quality of care. He also teaches in the campus-wide interdisciplinary patient safety course with the other authors of this book. Dr. Fuji is a Patient Safety Expert Panel Reviewer for the Creighton Center for Health Services Research and Patient Safety, Patient Safety Organization.

Kimberly A. Galt, RPh, PharmD, FASHP

Kimberly Galt is the director of the Creighton Center for Health Services Research and Patient Safety, the associate dean for research in the School of Pharmacy and Health Professions, and a professor at Creighton University. Her research has emphasized identification of errors, error reduction, and error prevention for patients and healthcare providers to achieve both safety and quality in patient care. She has contributed to understanding the human-technology safety issues as emerging health information technologies have gained use in health care. Dr. Galt has served on several study sections for the Agency for Healthcare Research and Quality, chairs the eHealth Council for the state of Nebraska, and chaired the interprofessional task force on patient safety curriculum development for Creighton University. She, along with the coauthors of this book, has been teaching the campus-wide interdisciplinary patient safety course since 2005. Dr. Galt is a Patient Safety Expert Panel Reviewer for the Creighton Center for Health Services Research and Patient Safety, Patient Safety Organization.

John M. Gleason, DBA

John M. Gleason is a professor emeritus of Decision Sciences, Department of Information Systems and Technology, College of Business Administration, Creighton University. He has taught graduate and undergraduate courses in operations research, decision sciences, and environmental risk analysis in business, engineering, and environmental science programs at several universities. Dr. Gleason has served as a member of the Editorial Advisory Board of *RISK: Health, Safety & Environment*, is a past vice president of the Risk Assessment & Policy Association, and is the recipient of government, professional society, and university research honors and awards. His research interests include operations research, decision technologies, and risk analysis, with his recent research concentrating on the theory and application of data envelopment analysis. His focus in this book is on decision analysis, technology, and systems analysis issues related to patient safety.

Janet K. Graves, PhD, RN

Janet Graves is the chair of the Traditional Curriculum at Creighton University School of Nursing. She taught Nursing of Children for several years and currently teaches Informatics in Health Care. Her interest in patient safety developed when providing nursing care for children. Her current work in informatics has led to interest in information technologies that have the potential to improve patient safety. Dr. Graves is also the director of eLearning in the School of Nursing. Her research interests include uses of mobile information devices at the point of care and effective methods of online teaching and learning.

Barbara M. Harris, MSW, PhD

Barbara Harris is the field practicum coordinator for the Department of Social Work at Creighton University. She teaches practice courses in social work. Her community involvement is primarily focused on family violence and child poverty. She served on several community boards to identify the intraprofessional approaches to addressing social welfare needs. As director of the Center for the Study of Children's Issues and as a founding member of the Domestic Violence Coordinating Council, she advanced this interprofessional framework. She served on the interprofessional task force on patient safety curriculum development for Creighton University. She, along with the coauthors of this book, developed the interdisciplinary patient safety course in 2005.

Pat Hoidal, RN, MPH, CPHQ

Pat Hoidal is the director of Performance Improvement and Risk Management at Saint Elizabeth Regional Medical Center in Lincoln, Nebraska. As the patient safety officer, she is responsible for facilitating the use of evidence-based practice and process improvement tools. She currently leads initiatives aimed at improving patient safety and quality of care by the use of the GE WorkOut and TeamSTEPPS models. She is a member of the administrative Quality and Patient Safety Council and has been involved in a variety of clinical quality improvement efforts for the medical center. Prior to coming to Saint Elizabeth, Hoidal spent seven years with Creighton University Medical Center. While at Creighton, Hoidal served as director of Quality and Patient Safety, and Risk Management. She led initiatives to implement The Joint Commission's National Patient Safety Goals and conducted root cause analysis and failure-mode analysis to address system issues related to patient safety. A graduate of the University of Nebraska with a degree in Nursing, Hoidal received her MPH degree from the University of Minnesota. She performed research on the relationship of personality characteristics to job performance and has published on nursing competency assessment.

Catherine Mahern, JD

Catherine Mahern is an associate professor of law at Creighton University, where she is the Director of Clinic Programs and the holder of the Kearney Chair in Clinical Legal Education. Her work focuses on legal education and the acquisition of lawyering skills. Professor Mahern has served on several committees on the improvement of justice and access to the profession, including the Nebraska Supreme Court's Implementation Committee on Pro Se Litigation and the Minority and Justice Implementation Committee.

Robert J. McQuillan, MD—In Memoriam

Dr. McQuillan was an associate professor and chair, Department of Anesthesiology at the Creighton University Medical Center and Creighton University School of Medicine. Dr. McQuillan completed his Doctor of Medicine at Creighton University and his anesthesiology residency with a fellowship in pain medicine at the University of Missouri–Kansas City/St. Luke's Hospital. He provided strong interprofessional leadership to bring crew resource management techniques, including the Agency for Healthcare Research and Quality TeamSTEPPS program, into the operating room and presurgical and postsurgical care models. He conducted his work at Creighton University Medical Center and nationally, leading interdisciplinary education and research on the implementation and evaluation of the effectiveness of this approach to patient safety. He continuously studied human factors science with a goal of improving patient safety, motivated to care for those patients who received his services in the operating room. Dr. McQuillan was a founding faculty member of the campus-wide interdisciplinary Foundations in

Patient Safety course at Creighton University. His sense of purpose, enthusiasm, and commitment to improving patient safety will be remembered among his colleagues and his patients.

Keli Mu, PhD, OTR/L

Keli Mu is an associate professor and vice chair of Occupational Therapy in the School of Pharmacy and Health Professions at Creighton University. Dr. Mu's research interests include occupational therapy and physical therapy practice errors and patient safety, program evaluation, evidence-based practice, and issues related to professional education. Dr. Mu has led or coled several research projects focusing on practice errors and patient safety. In 2004, he received the James S. Todd Memorial Award from the National Patient Safety Foundation for his patient safety research. As one of the coauthors for this book, he has taught in the campus-wide interprofessional patient safety course at Creighton University. Dr. Mu is a Patient Safety Expert Panel Reviewer for the Creighton Center for Health Services Research and Patient Safety, Patient Safety Organization.

Karen A. Paschal, PT, DPT, MS

Karen Paschal is an associate professor in the Department of Physical Therapy and a faculty member of the Creighton Center for Health Services Research and Patient Safety at Creighton University. Her research focuses on the adoption and use of health information technology across the healthcare delivery system. She serves on the Nebraska eHealth Council Health Information Security and Privacy Work Group and cochairs the education subcommittee. As chair of the physical therapy curriculum committee, she served on the Office of Interprofessional Education Advisory Committee and was a member of the Task Force on Patient Safety Curriculum responsible for designing, implementing, and evaluating a campus-wide course on patient safety. She has served as a consultant to educational programs in the area of curriculum development and assessment and serves on the Commission on Accreditation in Physical Therapy Education. Dr. Paschal is a Patient Safety Expert Panel Reviewer for the Creighton Center for Health Services Research and Patient Safety, Patient Safety Organization.

Ann M. Rule, PharmD

During the manuscript preparation, Ann Rule was a clinical assistant professor of Pharmacy Practice, School of Pharmacy and Health Professions, and Research Fellow at the Creighton University Center for Health Services Research and Patient Safety. Her prior experience includes 30 years of pharmacy practice in a variety of settings. During her fellowship, she was involved with Dr. Galt's grant with the Agency for Health Research and Quality on medication safety. This project involved the management of a field research study of 80 physicians in 32 office-based practices to determine the impact of PDA hand-held technologies on medication errors in prescribing. Dr. Rule was a member of Creighton's inter-professional task force on patient safety curriculum development and helped teach the interdisciplinary patient safety course. Dr. Rule is currently Director, Medical Liaison at Purdue Pharma L.P. and is based in Newark, Delaware.

Linda S. Scheirton, PhD

Linda Scheirton is the associate dean for Academic Affairs in the School of Pharmacy and Health Professions at Creighton University. She is coordinator of the Patient Safety Organization for Creighton Center for Health Services Research and Patient Safety and a faculty associate in the Center for Health Policy and Ethics. She has focused expertise in the moral management of patient error: disclosure, apology, and reparation. Current research efforts include the study of practitioner errors in occupational therapy and physical therapy practice as well as interest in patient safety issues in dentistry. Dr. Scheirton is a Patient Safety Expert Panel Reviewer for the Creighton Center for Health Services Research and Patient Safety, Patient Safety Organization.

CHAPTER 1

Key Concepts in Patient Safety

Kimberly A. Galt, Karen A. Paschal, and John M. Gleason

PURPOSE

The purpose of this chapter is to provide all health professionals with the core theory and knowledge they need to understand and practice patient care using patient safety principles. This core knowledge underpins and supports the remaining chapters and case studies. Every chapter that follows incorporates these safety principles.

OBJECTIVES

After completing this chapter, you will be able to:
- Define the scope of the problem of unsafe healthcare practices in the United States
- Compare and contrast the individual patient and public viewpoint about healthcare safety and harm
- Describe the historical development of the theories and practices of safety in industries other than health care
- Describe the rationale for professionals to integrate basic concepts of patient safety in health care
- Use the basic terminology and vocabulary of patient safety in health care

VIGNETTE

I watched my father in the hospital bed. He was trying to rise, but his muscles were so weak that he could not sit up on his own. Although the staff had taught him to roll over on his side and push up, he could no longer lift his upper body with his arms. What happened to him? I was only 13 years old at the time. My dad had been in the hospital for over 2 years but still kept losing weight. The doctors could not find the correct diagnosis. When entering the hospital, he was a tall man of 6'4" who weighed 195 pounds, but he weighed only 125 pounds at discharge. He was tested for all kinds of cancer and was referred for extensive psychological testing. He was accused of starving himself. He had supervised feedings and extensive counseling. Self-insured as a small business owner, my father's resources were drained, and there was no way to continue to pay for services. On the day that he was discharged, a medical bill for $350,000 was handed to my mom. Dad's hair was sparse and his eye color faded. He was starving to death. He went home expecting to die. My mom started reading on her own. She learned about a problem with gluten absorption. Later we made a diagnosis of celiac disease. She took action and obtained help.

Five years later, I learned about parenteral nutrition in pharmacy school. Why was Dad's nutrition not maintained by this means? Missed diagnoses—they must be common. How could 2 years of testing overlook what my mom could find? My father was now a man with permanent neurologic disabilities secondary to severe malnutrition, and my family was financially insolvent. After money was no longer available, Dad was abandoned. For what were all of those resources used? The impact of unsafe health care caused by a medical error is very real to my family.

SAFETY AS A FOUNDATION OF HIGH-QUALITY HEALTH CARE

The safety of a patient depends on each health professional's ability to "do the right thing." As a health professional continuously works at improving quality, individual performance shifts to "doing the right thing well."[1] Assuring the safety of the patient to whom services are provided is an essential dimension of professional performance. The Institute of Medicine (IOM) published a report in 2000 entitled *To Err is Human: Building a Safer Health System*.[2] This report describes the risks of medical care in the United States and the documented harm that has occurred because of unsafe practices in the healthcare systems.[i] What is a safe patient practice? A patient safety practice is a type of process or structure whose application reduces the probability of adverse events resulting from exposure to the healthcare system across a range of diseases and procedures.[1] The care we deliver and the way we deliver it should have the least potential to cause patient harm and the greatest potential to result in an optimal outcome for the patient. Patients assume that this is what we do when we take care of them.

THE CASE FOR IMPROVING PATIENT SAFETY

Unsafe Practices: The Scope of the Problem of Errors in Health Care

The IOM has summarized the evidence about medical errors in the United States. This evidence estimates that up to 98,000 individuals die every year in hospitals as a result of medical errors and that 2% of hospitalized patients experience a preventable adverse event. Sufficient numbers of these events result in serious harm.[2] Examples of the most common errors include improper transfusions, surgical injuries and wrong-site surgery, suicides, restraint-related injuries or death, falls, burns, pressure ulcers, misdiagnoses, and mistaken patient identities. Some of the most frequent errors occur in the most intensive care environments, such as emergency rooms, operating rooms, and intensive care units. On the other hand, the majority of care is provided in outpatient and ambulatory areas, an environment that has been described as a nonsystem. Care is provided without complete access to medical information about patients; often multiple providers serve different aspects of a patient's care needs, and the emphasis on accountability and reporting is nearly nonexistent.

The medical liability system is also regarded as a major disincentive to open disclosure of information about errors. The impact has been to discourage the

---

[i] More recent reports have been published that inform us further about additional and emerging problems in safety and our progress in addressing these causes. For example, a 2006 report entitled *Medication Errors by the Committee on Identifying and Preventing Medication Errors Board on Health Care Services* was released. It focuses more deeply on problems with medications. These reports can be accessed through the Institute of Medicine website (http://www.iom.edu/). A lifelong practice of staying informed as these sentinel reports are published is vital to maintaining professional knowledge and evolving science and evidence in patient safety and professional practice.

systematic study of uncovering causes and learning how to change what we do from our errors. Many healthcare providers fear costly law suits or loss of employment and other harm that can occur to those who are involved in errors or unsafe practices. Many anecdotal reports of employment termination exist because of an individual's unfortunate involvement in a medical error. In a recent study of employees who work in physicians' offices, 24% of the offices reported that an individual has been dismissed from employment because of a medical error that occurred in that office. Not surprisingly, only 65% of the offices reported that they can openly discuss errors.[3] The lack of cooperation and perceived risk of disclosure discourage healthcare providers, organizations, and payers, often third party, from openly discussing and investing in the improvements needed to achieve a safer, higher quality healthcare environment.

The Real Problem Is Harm, Not Errors

The harm that occurs is impressive when the financial, resource utilization, and healthcare system impact is evaluated; however, the immeasurable costs are reflected in the life experiences of the patients who are harmed and their loved ones and friends. This is clear in the stories of our authors. Fear and distrust of the health system and the individual health professionals who serve emerge as the dominant belief system for patients. The repercussions of harm are both physical and psychological. Often there is no reversing of the damages. The permanency of injuries is a constant reminder of the harm. A health professional's confidence, enthusiasm, and desire to serve in this capacity are explicitly challenged when dealing with these situations. Thus, this touches everyone.

Who Is to Blame?

This common question always arises after an error occurs. It strikes fear, guilt, anger, and the desire for restitution or even revenge from some. These feelings emerge in both patients and family members, as well as in the professionals involved. It is too easy to blame an individual, such as a healthcare provider or health system employee, making the one person wholly responsible for the *complex and often inadequate health system* in which most of us work. The lack of integration of clinical decision support systems, the paucity of training in patient safety for professionals, and the lack of organizational leadership to achieve safer systems all contribute to each of the errors that get reported.

Further compounding this challenge is the cultural and social context. After harm occurs, the individuals directly involved become isolated. Because the unsafe event usually happens to one person, one episode at a time, a critical mass of persons who are simultaneously having the experience does not exist. Socially, this means that individuals who are harmed have difficulty with advocacy because there is generally a lack of understanding at the local level among those they interact with about the nature and prevalence of this problem. Healthcare professionals need to know much more about how patients, consumers of health care, react and cope to achieve a resolution.

The Science of Safety: What We Have Learned from Engineering, Aviation, and Nuclear Power

Healthcare professionals are relative newcomers to the science of safety and errors, or accidents. We have the privilege of being able to draw on a knowledge base developed in the engineering disciplines, a knowledge base that continues to expand as a result of unfortunate catastrophes (e.g., Bopal and Chernobyl) or near catastrophes (Three Mile Island). Such incidents with high-risk technologies suggest that planned safety measures are not sufficient to eliminate continuing safety threats and further accidents. For a better understanding of accidents related to high-risk technologies, read the seminal book *Normal Accidents* by sociologist Charles Perrow.[4]

RISKY SYSTEMS AND NORMAL ACCIDENTS

The ineffectiveness of planned safety measures is a result of the complicated nature of most "risky" systems. In such cases, there are an unimaginable number of ways in which "two or more failures (can occur) among components that interact in some unexpected way."[4, p.4] Perrow refers to this as the "interactive complexity" of a system.

Failures resulting from interactive complexity, however, typically become significant safety threats only when the system is "tightly coupled."[4] If neither the time nor a means to appropriately intervene exists after an "interactive complexity" failure, then potentially catastrophic events may ensue. Perrow notes that the system characteristics of interactive complexity and tight coupling can be expected to result in an accident, and he refers to such as "normal accidents."

Over the years, for example, the air traffic control system has been modified in numerous ways to avoid normal accidents. Some of us may remember flying in circles (sometimes for hours) at various airports as a result of weather disturbances that delayed arrivals and departures. The safety/accident risks of tracking and controlling planes stacked in various layers over an airport are evident. This danger no longer exists. Now, when weather events warrant, departures are delayed at the origin airport. Airspace density at the destination airport affected by the weather is reduced. Planes are no longer stacked at the destination, and passengers fume in airport lounges rather than in the air. Most observers would agree that the air traffic control system has been improved as a result of efforts to reduce interactive complexity and tight coupling.

Regardless of efforts to reduce normal accidents in many engineering environments, they continue to occur, and the blame for such accidents continues to be diffused. For example, the President's Commission to Investigate the Accident at Three Mile Island distributed blame rather diffusely but placed primary blame on the operators. Metropolitan Edison, on the other hand, blamed the equipment. A study conducted for the Nuclear Regulatory Commission blamed systems design.[4]

In all cases, however, healthcare professionals prefer to avoid the necessity of placing blame. Instead, we would rather an incident not occur at all. This is the focus of this book. How can the healthcare system improve in order to avoid errors, mistakes, and accidents and better ensure patient safety? How do healthcare professionals continuously assure this? Healthcare delivery systems are complex and dynamic. New technologies, care approaches, and evidence are constantly emerging. Thus, we must learn how the science of safety should be applied regularly and continuously in our practices. Given the experience that the engineering disciplines have gained in industries such as aviation and nuclear energy, we should evidently focus on system issues such as interactive complexity and tight coupling in health care.

For example, if the interactive complexity of a system results in an error in prescribing or dispensing a routine medication to a patient hospitalized for elective surgery, the loose coupling of the system may ensure that the patient suffers no severe consequences. In this instance, system redundancies have time to become active. The error may be caught by a nurse reviewing the patient's records before administering the medication to the patient, or the patient may notice that the color/shape of the medication is inconsistent with that which is routinely taken. On the other hand, if interactive complexities lead to an error in a trauma center, a place of care delivery where many rapid and near instantaneous care decisions are made, there may be neither the time nor the means to recover from the error appropriately, and the patient may suffer irreparable harm. Thus, the risks in the latter case are more significant than in the former.

RISK ANALYSIS, PUBLIC POLICY, AND REGULATION

As healthcare professionals strive to improve patient safety, issues such as risk analysis, public policy, and regulation must be considered. Implications of these topics for a variety of disciplines, including health and safety, can be found in journals such as *Risk Analysis* and *RISK: Health, Safety & Environment*, the journals of the Society for Risk Analysis and the Risk Assessment and Policy Association, respectively. For example, risk analysts have questioned the efficacy of public policy and regulation, which require huge expenditures for a small reduction in one type of risk, when similar expenditures could yield significant reductions in other types of risks. With respect to patient safety, the identification of potential risks and the costs of mitigating those risks need to be considered in order to prioritize patient safety efforts.

Emerging evidence and practical applications in health care have recently become available in application-oriented publications, web-based resources, and other media resources. Two recently emerging journals that focus on safety in health care are the *Journal of Quality and Patient Safety*, published by the Joint Commission on Accreditation of Healthcare Organizations, and the *Journal of Patient Safety*.

We also need to recognize that risk perceptions of the lay public are relevant to efforts to improve patient safety. Evidence suggests that the public uses error rates to judge the quality of health care and that information gained from the Internet may complicate public perceptions.[5,6] The federal government is increasing attention on the potential for centralized reporting of unsafe events. A system for this, similar to the system that exists for aviation reporting, will likely emerge in the next few years.

Considerable research has been devoted to measuring public perceptions of an assortment of health, safety, and environmental risks. Various risk paradigms have emerged from both quantitative and qualitative research, including engineering, psychological, and cultural paradigms. Evidence shows that psychometric models (based on statistical techniques such as factor analysis and principal components analysis) may be more useful than cultural models in explaining variances in risk perception. Moreover, considerable differences exist between the level of risks that experts perceive and those the lay public perceives, and the latter group tends to use a variety of (perhaps unreliable) heuristic processes in estimating risk. If there is truth to the adage that "perception is reality," then those who are attempting to reduce risks to patient safety and health must have an appropriate understanding of relevant risks as well as an understanding of the heuristic processes that the public uses in risk estimation. Moreover, because risk mitigation is costly, the value of a clear understanding of statistical methods and statistical decision analysis in scientific risk analysis is evident.

Although healthcare professionals may not individually be a master of the use of these tools, we all have a responsibility to understand and use the best practices and approaches that emerge from these scientific analyses as they are revealed.

IMPORTANT GOVERNANCE AND ORGANIZATIONS IN PATIENT SAFETY

Different groups have formed in the government, private healthcare sector, professions, and consumers to advance the causes, concerns, and solutions to the problems of patient safety. These groups have emerged from a true social need to improve the situation. Some of these organizations are oriented toward providing access to the newest information that may be useful in advancing safety. Others provide resources and funding to study difficult or newly emerging problems in safety. Political activism for regulatory, legislative, and policy change is central to some. The Appendix at the end of this chapter provides a comprehensive listing of groups whose missions and purposes are associated with the area of patient safety. You are encouraged to go to the Websites identified for these organizations to gain an appreciation and understanding of the mission and purpose of each.

BASIC CONCEPTS OF PATIENT SAFETY

The Principles and Tenets of Patient Safety

As stated in the IOM report: "Whether a person is sick or just trying to stay healthy, they should not have to worry about being harmed by the health system itself."[2] There are some key principles and tenets that serve to motivate healthcare providers to continuously improve efforts in patient safety:

- Healthcare professionals are intrinsically motivated to improve patient safety because of the ethical foundation, professional norms, and expectations of our respective disciplines.
- Organizational leaders are responsible for setting the standards for achieving safety at the highest level and will do so in response to societal expectations.
- Consumers are becoming increasingly aware of the healthcare safety problem and are not accepting of it.[7]
- There is substantial room for improvement of healthcare systems and practices that will result in a reduction in both error potential and harm.

To improve safety, healthcare professionals must recognize the characteristics that can make this effort a success. First, we must be able to collect data on errors and incidents within the local organization in order to identify opportunities for improvements and to be able to track progress. Second, we must develop an organizational culture that is founded on the concept of safety. Third, complex processes must be analyzed using appropriate tools. Finally, as much standardization as is possible should be accomplished while still allowing individuals the independent authority to solve encountered problems in a creative way.

Safety and Quality Are Concepts on a Continuum

It is a challenge to understand the concepts of safety and quality. According to the IOM report, these are inseparable. When does the concept of safety end and the concept of quality begin? In essence, when our care is safe, we do no harm and have the lowest potential to do harm through the processes we use and the practices we adopt. When we provide the highest quality of care, we make choices and deliver care that has the greatest potential to achieve the best outcome possible for our patients.

By merging the two concepts, opportunity costs are created. It costs something to assure safety. Healthcare providers must assess opportunity costs to understand the *true cost* of any course of action. If we ignore opportunity costs, we may produce the illusion that the benefits of achieving the highest standards of safety cost nothing at all. These unseen opportunity costs are *hidden costs* incurred. Although it is sometimes hard to compare the benefits and losses of alternative courses of action, it is not necessarily so difficult in patient safety. For example, if we want to reduce the number of opportunities that the wrong medicine is dispensed by the pharmacist before it is given to the patient, we must take the time to check the manufacturer's medication container against the medicines that we place into the prescription container for the patient. This process takes time and employees all get paid a salary. If we were to employ too few people, the cost would be increased by potential medication dispensing errors reaching the patient. Add to this another patient care step, counseling. When pharmacists counsel patients directly about their medications before dispensing them, 89% of product-dispensing errors are caught before reaching the patient.[8] If we do not adequately staff the pharmacy, such that pharmacists do not have time to counsel patients in a thorough manner, the number of medication errors that reach the patient increases dramatically.

One way to identify opportunities to improve safety is to apply the practices of continuous quality improvement, a method widely used in many industries, including health care.[9] Our challenge is to apply this practice from a patient-centered perspective.

TAXONOMY, DEFINITIONS, AND TERMS

What Is a Taxonomy?

Taxonomies are the systematic arrangement of entities in any field into categories or classes based on common characteristics such as properties, morphology, and subject matter. In other words, a taxonomy organizes our ideas into relationships that have meaning. Taxonomies are global, professional, and sometimes practice-setting specific.

Why Is a Taxonomy Important in Patient Safety?

System improvement is the major way in which patients will be safer when receiving health care. Much of system improvement requires our ability to count the number and types of events or occurrences that are indicators of what we are trying to affect or change. Without a common taxonomy, which is our current system, we will not be able to keep track of events to measure change. A common language is also necessary between healthcare providers and organizational and system employees. We all need to understand patient safety concepts with the same meaningfulness; therefore, your charge is to understand the patient safety taxonomy in the context of your workplace, its improvement efforts, and the patients you serve.

In patient safety, some key terms and definitions should be understood. Particularly when healthcare providers are working between and within different professional backgrounds, we must have a common understanding of definitions and terms used in patient safety. Definitions are of vital importance when they are used to describe measurements and attributes. In the case of patient safety, there is a great need to count events and determine the magnitude of impact of events. The core terms that are essential to know and understand are highlighted here. In addition, a more complete listing is included in the Taxonomy of Terms and the Source section of the textbook. A working knowledge of the terms and concepts shown here should be acquired:

> *Accident*—an event that involves damage to a defined system that disrupts the ongoing or future output of the system.[2] Accident is another word for the event itself and not the causes that supersede it.
>
> *Adverse event*—an injury resulting from a medical intervention.[2] Adverse events may occur because of error or because of an intrinsic negative reaction not related to error. Adverse events may come about because of both error and nonerror causes. For example, a patient may have an adverse drug event. This may occur because the patient could not tolerate the particular chemical structure of the drug and as a result experienced a harmful effect.

Error—failure of a planned action to be completed as intended or use of a wrong plan to achieve an aim; the accumulation of errors results in accidents. Errors can include problems in practice, products, procedures, and systems.[2] There are different types of errors. The taxonomy describing error is in the context of systems.

Active error—an error that occurs at the level of the front-line operator and whose effects are felt almost immediately.[2]

Latent error—errors in the design, organization, training, or maintenance that lead to operator errors and whose effects typically lie dormant in the system for lengthy periods of time.[2]

Human factors—study of the interrelationships between humans, the tools they use, and the environment in which they live and work.[2] Human factors testing and evaluation is a field of methodologies to assess the effectiveness and suitability of any human–system interface.[10]

Patient safety—freedom from accidental injury; ensuring patient safety involves the establishment of operational systems and processes that minimize the likelihood of errors and maximize the likelihood of intercepting them when they occur.[2] The concept of patient safety includes both responding to and preventing errors.

Patient safety practice—a type of process or structure whose application reduces the probability of adverse events resulting from exposure to the health system across a range of conditions or procedures.[11]

Quality of care—the degree to which health services for individuals and populations increase the likelihood of desired health outcomes and are consistent with current professional knowledge.[2] Donabedian points out that depending on where we are located in the system of care and the nature and extent of our responsibilities, several formulations of quality are legitimate. In general, quality of care is inclusive of care by practitioners and other providers, care received by the patient, and care received by the community. These are levels of care that can be assessed for quality.[12]

Standard—a minimum level of acceptable performance or results, or excellent levels of performance, or the range of acceptable performance or results. The American Society for Testing and Materials defines six types of standards.[2]

1. Standard test method—a procedure for identifying, measuring, and evaluating a material, product, or system.
2. Standard specification—a statement of a set of requirements to be satisfied and the procedures to determine whether each of the requirements is satisfied.

3. Standard practice—a procedure for performing one or more specific operations or functions.
4. Standard terminology—a document comprising terms, definitions, descriptions, explanations, abbreviations, or acronyms.
5. Standard guide—a series of options or instructions that do not recommend a specific course of action.
6. Standard classification—a systematic arrangement or division of products, systems, or services into groups based on similar characteristics.

System—a set of interdependent elements interacting to achieve a common aim. These elements may be both human and nonhuman (equipment, technologies, etc.).[2] In health care, it is well recognized that all systems have a human–system interdependency and interface. In the patient safety work we do, we concentrate on system failures and improvements.

Microsystem—an organizational unit built around the definition of repeatable core service competencies. Elements of a microsystem include (1) a core team of healthcare professionals, (2) a defined population of patients, (3) carefully designed work processes, and (4) an environment capable of linking information on all aspects of work and patient or population outcomes to support ongoing evaluation of performance.[2]

SUMMARY

The scope of the problem of unsafe healthcare practices in the United States is large. The dynamic nature of health care further complicates the problem of safety. As new technologies and approaches to care are incorporated into the daily practice of health professionals, new opportunities for unsafe practices are created. By understanding the historical development of the theories and practices of safety in industries other than health care, we are better positioned in health care to incorporate improvements from these lessons learned. Thus, it is important for professionals to integrate basic concepts of patient safety into health care. We must know the basic terminology and vocabulary of patient safety in health care as a common language between us in our disciplines in order to incorporate patient safety practices that are understood and supported by all of us. The harm, fear, isolation, and eventual poor health outcome for patients as a result of unsafe practices are avoidable for most patients. If we incorporate the science of safety into our ongoing daily practices, we are sure to reduce the magnitude and extent of harm and injury that results for all of us.

A CLOSING CASE

Read the following case, and use the questions that follow to apply what you have learned in this chapter:

A.L. was in a rollover motor vehicle accident while traveling 3 hours from her home early one weekend morning. She was removed from the vehicle by paramedics and transported by ambulance to the nearest regional hospital. In the emergency room, she was examined, received staples to close a head wound, and had radiographs taken. Although she was sore all over, her main complaint was pain and numbness in the middle of her shoulder that continued down her arm into her fingers. The radiographs were negative, and the patient was discharged from the hospital after 2 days of observation. She was to see her family physician to get the staples removed.

The patient's symptoms did not improve, and when she saw her family physician, she requested a referral to physical therapy. When her symptoms did not improve with physical therapy, the physical therapist discussed additional imaging studies with the patient's physician. Magnetic resonance imaging (MRI) revealed three fractures and a subluxation of the C6-C7 vertebrae, which would be consistent with the patient's symptoms. (The original plain films were blurry in this area.) Subsequently, A.L. underwent a cervical fusion. Although improvement was noted, she now has some restriction in her neck movements.

1. Describe the adverse event in this case.
2. Did an error occur? If so, what was it?
3. Was the patient harmed?
4. Who should be blamed?

Discussion Questions to Launch Further Investigation

For further investigation, seek answers to these questions. The following resource list may be helpful to you in this inquiry:

1. Distinguish between risk and harm. Why is it important to differentiate these two concepts?
2. Why do we need to openly discuss errors that occur in practice?
3. Why is it incorrect to hold one person solely responsible for an error that occurs and reaches a patient?

- Agency for Health care Research and Quality. Web M&M: Morbidity and Mortality Rounds on the Web. Available at: http://www.webmm.ahrq.gov/. Accessed September 8, 2008.
- *Making Health Care Safer: A Critical Analysis of Patient Safety Practices.* Evidence Report/Technology Assessment: Number 43. Rockville, MD: Agency for Healthcare Research and Quality, U.S. Department of Health and Human Services; July 20, 2001. AHRQ Publication No. 01-E-058.

REFERENCES

1. Shojania KG, Duncan BW, McDonald KM, Wachter RM. *Making Health Care Safer: A Critical Analysis of Patient Safety Practices.* Evidence report/technology assessment—Number 43. AHRQ Publication 01-E058 July 20, 2001.
2. Kohn LT, Corrigan JM, Donaldson MS, eds. *To Err Is Human: Building a Safer Health System.* Washington, DC: National Academy Press; 2000, p. 5.
3. Galt KA, Rule A, Clark BE, Bramble JD, Taylor W, Moores KG. Best practices in medication safety—areas for improvement in the primary care physician's office. In Henriksen K, Battles JB, Marks ES, Lewin DI, editors. *AHRQ Advances in Patient Safety: From Research to Implementation.* Vol.1, Research findings. AHRQ Publication No. 05-0021-1. Rockville, MD: Agency for Healthcare Research and Quality; Feb. 2005; 101–129.
4. Perrow C. *Normal Accidents.* Princeton, NJ: Princeton University Press; 1999.
5. Anonymous. Internet use affects health care decision making, survey confirms. *Am J Health Syst Pharm* 2001b;58:107–108.
6. Anonymous. Consumers use error rates to judge health care quality, survey shows. *Am J Health Syst Pharm* 2001a;58:103,106.
7. Kaiser Family Foundation. National Survey on Consumers' Experiences with Patient Safety and Quality Information. Available at: http://www.kff.org/kaiserpolls/pomr111704pkg.cfm. Accessed September 8, 2008.
8. Kuyper A. Patient counseling detects prescription errors. *Hosp Pharm* 1993;12:1180–1181, 1184–1189.
9. Leape LL. Errors in medicine. *JAMA* 1994;272(23):1851–1857.
10. Charleton SG, O'Brien TG. *Handbook of Human Factors Testing and Evaluation,* 2nd ed. London: Lawrence Erlbaum Associates; 2002.
11. Brennan TA, Leape LL, Laird NM, et al. Incidence of adverse events and negligence in hospitalized patients: results of the Harvard Medical Practice Study I. *N Engl J Med* 1991;324:370–376.
12. Donabedian A. The quality of care: how can it be assessed? In: Graham NO. *Quality in Health Care: Theory, Application and Evolution.* Gaithersburg, MD: Aspen Publishers; 1995:32–44.

Appendix

Patient Safety Relevant Organizations and Acronyms Guide

Agency for Health Care Policy and Research	AHCPR
Agency for Healthcare Research and Quality	AHRQ
American Hospital Association	AHA
American Medical Association	AMA
American National Standards Institute	ANSI
American Nurses Association	ANA
Area Health Education Center Program	AHEC
Association for the Advancement of Medical Instrumentation	AAMI
Aviation Safety Reporting System	ASRS
Center for Quality Improvement and Patient Safety	CQuIPS
Centers for Disease Control and Prevention	CDC
Centers for Education and Research on Therapeutics	CERTs
Conditions of Participation	CoP
Department of Defense	DoD
Department of Health and Human Services	DHHS
Department of Labor	DOL
Department of Veterans Affairs	VA
Diabetes Quality Improvement Project	DQIP
Employee Benefit Research Institute	EBRI
Employee Retirement Income Security Act	ERISA
Epidemic Intelligence Service	EIS
Federal Aviation Administration	FAA

(continued)

15

Patient Safety Relevant Organizations and Acronyms Guide (continued)

Federation of State Medical Boards	FSMB
Fiscal Year	FY
Food and Drug Administration	FDA
Health Care Financing Administration	HCFA
Health Resources and Services Administration	HRSA
Healthcare Cost and Utilization Project	HCUP
Indian Health Service	HIS
Institute of Medicine	IOM
Intensive care unit	ICU
Joint Commission on Accreditation of Healthcare Organizations	JCAHO
National Aeronautics and Space Administration	NASA
National Association of Insurance Commissioners	NAIC
National Business Coalition on Health	NBCH
National Committee for Quality Assurance	NCQA
National Coordinating Council for Medication Error Reporting and Prevention	NCCMERP
The National Forum for Health Care Quality Measurement and Reporting	Quality Forum
National Health Care Survey	NHCS
National Nosocomial Infections Surveillance	NNIS
National Patient Safety Foundation	NPSF
National Patient Safety Partnership	NPSP
National Practitioner Data Bank	NPDB
Occupational Safety and Health Administration	OSHA
Office of Personnel Management	OPM
Operating room	OR
Pension and Welfare Benefits Administration	PWBA
Quality Assessment/Performance Improvement	QAPI
Quality Interagency Coordination Task Force	QuIC
Study of Clinically Relevant Indicators for Pharmacologic Therapy	SCRIPT
Veterans Health Administration	VHA
Washington (DC) Business Group on Health	WBGH

Adapted from *Doing What Counts for Patient Safety: Federal Actions to Reduce Medical Errors and Their Impact.* Report of the Quality Interagency Coordination Task Force (QuIC) to the President, February 2000. Quality Interagency Coordination Task Force. Washington, DC. Available from: http://www.quic. gov/report/toc.htm.

Keeping the Patient Safe

Ann M. Rule, Karen A. Paschal, and Barbara M. Harris

PURPOSE

The purpose of this chapter is to understand safety from the individual patient's point of view. The patient's experience with health care, a "safe journey" (no aviation pun intended), including interactions with care providers, healthcare organizations, and their caregivers, is studied.

OBJECTIVES

After completing this chapter, you will be able to:

- Explain the patient's role of working with the healthcare team to insure medical safety
- Evaluate evidence-based safety practice recommendations that are patient-centered
- Describe gaps in the patient's healthcare that may lead to medical error
- Describe families' roles in relation to patient safety
- Describe caregivers' roles in relation to patient safety

VIGNETTE

"You just don't make a mistake like that on someone's kid. They're supposed to be professionals." These are the words of a grief-stricken father whose infant daughter died after the administration of a dose of heparin that was 1,000 times stronger than it should have been. She was one of six premature babies who were accidentally given adult doses of this anticlotting drug in an Indianapolis hospital in 2006; three of the babies died. Each of the children was to receive a 10-unit dose, but instead received 10,000 units.[1] Both vials had "similar blue labels and a common shape." After the deaths, the manufacturer "issued a safety alert to healthcare providers, but those blue labels remained on the drug."[2]

In 2007, a year later, a similar story appeared in the *Los Angeles Times*. This time, three children had their intravenous catheters flushed with heparin at a concentration 1,000 times higher than a normal dose. Fortunately, none of these children suffered adverse effects.[3] After this incident, the manufacturer changed its heparin packaging by adding a red caution label that must be torn off before the vial can be opened."[2]

Changes in packaging did not alleviate errors with heparin. A "mixing error" was the reported cause of a mistake that resulted in the administration of overdoses of heparin to 14 babies in a Corpus Christi, Texas, hospital in 2008. Two of those babies died.[4]

What can be done to make hospitals a safer place for newborns? What procedures can be put into place to prevent these errors from happening?

PATIENT SAFETY IN HEALTH CARE

When are patients safe? This can be understood by examining the different definitions that are put forth by organizations that are invested in reducing the problem of unsafe healthcare. The Institute of Medicine (IOM) defines patient safety as freedom from accidental injury. Ensuring patient safety involves the establishment of operational systems and processes that minimize the likelihood of errors and maximize the likelihood of intercepting them when they occur.[5] The National Patient Safety Foundation defines patient safety as the avoidance, prevention, and amelioration of adverse outcomes or injuries stemming from the process of healthcare. These events include errors, deviations, and accidents. Safety emerges from the interaction of the components. Patient safety is a subset of healthcare quality.[6] The Agency for Healthcare Research and Quality defines it as a type of process or structure in which the application reduces the probability of adverse events resulting from exposure to the healthcare system across a range of diseases and procedures.[7] It is clear that these definitions share many of the same components: improving systems or processes to minimize and/or prevent errors and thus harm. How to accomplish this is less clear, however. Ultimately, preventing our patients from suffering harm matters most. In order to achieve this, systems and processes must be in place not only to recognize actual errors but also to identify and prevent potential errors.

The IOM report *To Err Is Human* was published in 2000. It generated an enormous response from both the medical community and the public. Interestingly, a widespread difference exists in the perception of medical error by physicians and the public. Blendon et al. reported that 35% of physicians and 42% of the public reported experiencing errors in their own or a family member's care, but neither group viewed medical errors as a major issue in healthcare today. Both the physicians and the public believed that the number of preventable in-hospital deaths was lower than reported by the IOM.[8]

Patients may also base the quality of their healthcare on the quality of the interpersonal relationship they have with their healthcare providers. Patients may perceive they are safe if they view their healthcare providers as competent, caring, and trustworthy. Although these are certainly characteristics of a good healthcare provider, they do not replace systems and processes that are part of the culture of safety.

PATIENT'S BILL OF RIGHTS

Several organizations have developed and publicized a patient's bill of rights. Perhaps the most notable is the document developed by the American Hospital Association (see Table 2–1). Patient rights are described in a brochure entitled *The Patient Care Partnership: Understanding Expectations, Rights and Responsibilities.*[9] Of particular note is the inclusion of concomitant patient responsibilities. Do patients know they share responsibility for their health care? Have we done an effective job educating our patients about what those responsibilities are? Empowering patients to participate in their own care is especially challenging for several special populations. Older patients may have a particularly hard time with this concept as they grew up in an era when the physician told the patient what to do and physicians were never questioned. This form of deferent respect carries over to other health professionals as well. A common comment from older patients is, "Well, he's the doctor, he should know." Pediatric patients offer a different challenge. Children need adults to help them understand what to expect and to

Table 2–1 Websites with Recommendations for Patients

Healthcare Safety

Name	URL	Source
Patient Fact Sheet	http://www.ahrq.gov/consumer/20tips.htm	Agency for Healthcare Research and Quality
Medical Errors: Tips to Prevent Them	http://familydoctor.org/x2394.xml	American Academy of Family Physicians
What You Can Do to Make Health Care Safer	http://www.npsf.org/download/WhatYouCanDo.pdf	National Patient Safety Foundation
Preventing Infections in the Hospital—What You Can Do	http://www.npsf.org/paf/i/	National Patient Safety Foundation

Medication Safety

Name	URL	Description
"Your Role in Safe Medication Use, a Guide for Patients and Families"	http://www.macoalition.org/publicationsConsumerGuide.pdf	The Massachusetts Coalition for the Prevention of Medical Errors
Doctors Office Medication Safety Alert	http://www.ismp.org/Newsletters/consumer/alerts/StartinOffice.asp	Institute for Safe Medication Practices
Be an Informed Consumer	http://www.ismp.org/consumers/brochure.asp	Institute for Safe Medication Practices
Cancer Treatment Medication Safety Alert	http://www.ismp.org/Newsletters/acutecare/articles/cancertreatment.asp	Institute for Safe Medication Practices
Pharmacy Safety and Service—What You Should Expect	http://www.npsf.org/download/PharmacySafety.pdf	National Patient Safety Foundation

Patient Rights and Responsibilities

| Patient Safety and You | http://www.acponline.org/ptsafety/patientinfo.pdf | American College of Physicians |
| Patient Care Partnership | http://www.aha.org/aha/issues/Communicating-With-Patients/pt-care-partnership.html | American Hospital Association |

Patient Advocacy

| Role of the Patient Advocate | http://www.npsf.org/download/PatientAdvocate.pdf | National Patient Safety Foundation |

garner critical information from them as care decisions are made and care is provided. These two groups are examples of patients whom we often describe as *vulnerable*. This vulnerability refers to the patient's relatively high dependence on healthcare professionals to suggest the best approaches and protect them from harm and injury.

THE PATIENT EXPERIENCES GAPS IN CONTINUITY OF CARE

Common gaps in continuity of healthcare delivery present an enormous risk for error. Hospitals and health systems continue to struggle to decrease the number of gaps in the continuum of care. Recently, medication reconciliation has become a topic of discussion among the nation's top healthcare leaders. Medication reconciliation is a process to reduce errors and harm associated with medication issues as patients transfer from one level of care to another. This is observed as an inaccurate or incomplete transfer of the information about the patient's medication history and use from the patient to the health professionals when the patient is admitted to a hospital or other care facility or when a patient moves from the intensive care unit to a general care area of the hospital or when he or she leaves the hospital. This is just one of many examples of the numerous gaps that can occur in the continuum of care.[10–12] Let us explore this particular example further.

Patients who are admitted to the hospital are asked by the admitting nurse what medications they are currently taking. Sometimes patients are asked to bring their medication bottles with them. Unfortunately, not all patients are able to remember what they take, and thus, the information that they give is inaccurate. The admitting physician may have a written record of medications that have been prescribed for the patient, but it may be difficult to determine whether the patient has had the prescription filled or whether the patient is taking the medication as prescribed.

A study by Bedell et al. examined patients' medication bottles and their reported use of medications and compared these finding with the patients' medical records. Discrepancies in what physicians prescribed and what patients were actually taking were present in the majority of cases examined (76%). These discrepancies involved all classes of medications and included patients taking medications that were not recorded, patients not taking a recorded medication, and differences in dosing.[13]

Patients discharged from the hospital receive written instructions for taking medications as well as additional prescriptions if needed; however, after the patient gets home, he or she has to decide whether to continue his or her old medications or take only the medications listed on the discharge sheet. This can be quite confusing for patients, as trade names and generic names are used and hospital formularies may dictate what medication a patient may use. For example, a hospital has Protonix® as the preferred proton pump inhibitor; the patient is switched to that while in the hospital. At home, he takes Prilosec®. At discharge, his instructions are for Protonix®, but he also continues his Prilosec® because he does not know they are the same type of medicine.

Other gaps in continuity of health care include incomplete or inaccurate transfer of care information to another agency, such as a transfer from a hospital to a long-term care facility or home with a home healthcare company. In these situations, a plan of care and/or discharge instructions are sent to the receiving facility/agency, but important information may be missed. Another gap in continuity of care is observed at the time that a prescription(s) for medication is written and given to patients at discharge from a hospital. Without a discharge plan of care, the pharmacist is unable to do anything but simply fill the prescriptions. If pharmacists were given the plan of care, they would be able to evaluate more critically the medication therapy, educate patients, and reinforce the patients' instructions to optimize the patients' ability to self-treat with medicines and self-monitor their response to therapy.

The complexity of healthcare delivery in the 21st century has grown tremendously. Wachter and Shojana make the following statement in their book *Internal Bleeding*:

> All in all, while it is important for patients to do all they can to prevent fumbles from happening (we'll make some detailed recommendations in the final section of the book, but they include always carrying your list of current medications and asking what any new medication is for), the burden of making transitions smooth and error-free rests with the professionals and the systems at their disposal. When Marcus Welby did everything, handoffs were no big deal—there just weren't that many to make. Today, no single physician can do everything—or know everything—it takes to keep you and make you well. We can't go back to those good old days of the '50s, and, quite frankly, few patients or caregivers would want to try.
>
> Patients depend on us to steward the care process on their behalf. In the past, we have been far too laissez-faire about handoffs and far too resistant to standard procedures. We need stricter protocols and checklists for transitions. We need standard read-backs for critical voice exchanges. We need "bridge the gap" training for caregivers on both sides of a transfer—to make our hypothetical healthcare system less virtual, more real, and better integrated. We need to talk to each other not just after we make mistakes, but before they happen.[14, p.178–179.]

RELATIONSHIP BETWEEN THE PATIENT AND THE HEALTHCARE PRACTITIONER

The Healing Relationship

The Hippocratic Oath is well known. This ancient moral oath taken by physicians is associated with the obligation of healthcare practitioners to "do no harm" and is consistent with the image of an autonomous, authoritative practitioner. The patient rights movement in the 1970s, however, identified additional medical obligations.[15] The hallmark publication regarding medical morality and responsibility, *Principles of Biomedical Ethics*, was first published in 1979 by Tom Beauchamp and James Childress. Now in its fifth edition, this sentinel piece emphasizes the general acceptance of the norms of autonomy, beneficence, nonmaleficence, and justice.[16] These principles provide the framework for the healing relationship between a healthcare provider and his or her patient.

Pelegrino describes three elements in the health relationship: the fact of illness, the act of profession, and the act of medicine. Patients who are ill are vulnerable. They may be anxious, uncertain, fearful, or experiencing pain. As healthcare professionals, we offer our service to the patient, promising to help. This act of profession establishes the context for trust. The act of medicine is a response to the act of profession and is comprised of our examination, evaluation, and intervention for the betterment of the patient.[17] The patient places a special trust or confidence in the healthcare professional, who is then required to watch out for the best interests of the patient. By entering into this fiduciary relationship, *we* assume responsibility for safe patient care.

PATIENT EXPECTATIONS

Although the American public is aware that the healthcare environment is not always safe, the public's understanding of healthcare safety is limited. A survey by the National Patient Safety Foundation asked consumers, "What comes to mind when you think about patient safety issues in the healthcare environment?" Twenty-eight percent of respondents did not mention anything. Twenty percent mentioned exposure to infection. Thirteen percent cited the general level of care patients receive, and 11% cited qualification of health professionals. Consumers were also asked, "How have you learned about medical mistakes?" Most people learn about them through anecdotes. In fact, more than four of five respondents said that they knew about a situation in which a medical mistake was made. When asked how they heard about the most recent mistake, 42% cited a friend or relative; 39%, television, newspaper, or radio; and 12%, personal experience. Popular media coverage is generally limited to reporting anecdotal cases. This contributes to a "disconnect" between public perceptions and actual healthcare error rates.[18]

Consumers were asked to discern where healthcare mistakes are made by responding to the question, "When you think about the most recent medical mistake you know about, do you think of the mistake as occurring at the level of the healthcare system, at the organization level, or at the level of the healthcare provider?" Most people viewed errors as an "individual provider issue" rather than a failure in the process of delivering care in a complex delivery system. It is not surprising then to find these statements when asked about possible solutions to prevent medical mistakes: 75% of consumers believed that "keeping healthcare professionals with bad track records from providing care" and 69% believed that "better training of healthcare professionals" were the two most important solutions from their view.[18]

Improvement in patient safety is also hindered by the liability system. The threat of malpractice discourages the disclosure of medical errors. Legal proceedings encourage us to keep silent about errors committed and observed. Most errors and safety issues continue to go undetected and unreported, both externally and within healthcare organizations. This is a disincentive to improving safety through examining how to improve what we do. The irony of this is that most patients who have experienced harm do not want to pursue legal avenues as a method of resolution. The number-one desire of patients and family members who have experienced harm as a result of an unsafe practice is to protect others from experiencing it. Patients want us to learn from our mistakes and correct the underlying causes. We discuss this in more detail in Chapter 8.

PATIENTS' EXPERIENCES WITH SAFETY

Gone are the days when patients can be complacent about their healthcare. Healthcare has become so complex that patients must be involved in and strive to educate themselves about all aspects of their care. Encouraging patients to become an active member of their healthcare team reduces the risk of errors. A patient who is knowledgeable and vigilant may be able to identify potential risks for errors in their own or others' care. Patients should be encouraged to ask questions and make sure that they understand the answers and the implications.

What about the older patient who grew up thinking that the "doctor is always right" and was trained *not* to ask questions? This is a group of patients who particularly need a family member or friend to act as a patient advocate. As healthcare professionals, we can encourage and educate our patients to have this advocate participate and be present in the process of care delivery. Our influence on patients is great. For the vulnerable older population, this is giving them permission to be involved. For the child, this is a critical venue for gaining important care information and reducing harm as a result of inadequate communication.

ADVOCATES FOR THE PATIENT— SOMEONE TO WATCH OVER YOU

Today, patients admitted to hospitals are "sicker" and are discharged "quicker." Are today's patients capable of making the best medical decisions and spotting potential problems or errors with their care? Having a family member or friend serve as a patient advocate may help patients to participate more fully in their care and assume some of the responsibilities of their care, as discussed earlier. The National Patient Safety Foundation states that a patient advocate is someone who is a "supporter, believer, sponsor, promoter, campaigner, backer, or spokesperson." They suggest that the patient advocate be someone who the patient trusts, who can act assertively, and who knows the patient's feelings and beliefs.[19] Some hospitals and health systems have professional patient advocates that work with patients and families in their journey through the healthcare system.

SUMMARY

The patients we care for are unlikely to know of the risks inherent to the healthcare system. Patients need to be educated to take responsibility for assuring that the actions that are being taken in providing care to them are what they have agreed to and are expecting. Because of generational, cultural, and social norms, some patients may not feel that this responsibility can be acted on. You will need to invite it and give them permission to participate in their own care in this way. They must be encouraged and educated that they have a role in working with the healthcare team to insure medical safety. Because of gaps in healthcare delivery methods we use today, we should use evidence-based safety practice recommendations that are patient centered and also engage the patients' families and caregivers to take active roles in assuring their loved ones safety in care as well. This means that as healthcare professionals, we should anticipate more direct and frequent communication from patients, families, and caregivers in our daily professional practice.

A CLOSING CASE

Read the following case and use the questions that follow to apply what you have learned in this chapter:

Rose is a 79-year-old woman with hypertension, arthritis, diabetes, and chronic periodontal dental problems. She lives alone in a trailer in a rural county 40 miles away from a major city. She has no family and does not drive. Her 70-year-old neighbor, Fred, lives about 10 miles down the road and checks on Rose weekly. He takes Rose to doctor appointments and helps with weekly errands. Rose cooks, pays bills, and does light housekeeping. She especially enjoys the company of her television. She has difficulty hearing the telephone. She sits in a recliner 4 to 5 hours per day with the heels of her feet against the calf support of the recliner.

She received a check up from her physician a year ago. Rose scored 28/30 (minimal impairment) on the *Mini-Mental State Examination.*[20] At that time, she was diagnosed as having a stage II pressure sore on the dorsum of the right heel. The doctor reminded Rose to change positions often and to keep pressure off the heel. Rose did not keep her scheduled follow-up appointment with the doctor a month later.

Rose decided to apply elastic stockings (T.E.D. hose) last week (T.E.D. is a licensed trademark of TYCO International [U.S.]). The stockings were previously issued a year ago for management of lower-extremity edema. Because of joint pain in her hands and fingers associated with arthritis and difficulty applying the hose, she decided to leave the hose on. She slept in the hose for 7 days. This week Rose began to experience some discomfort in her foot with weight bearing. Fred stopped by to drop off the groceries and noticed some bleeding around the heel. Rose told Fred that she has been taking some Darvocet that she had left over from a dental abscess 3 years ago. She also complained of dizziness and fell in the bathroom yesterday. Fred decided that her problems were severe enough to take her to the emergency department at the local hospital. The T.E.D. hose were removed, and the wound was cultured. The culture revealed methicillin-resistant *Staphylococcus aureus* colonization. She was admitted to the hospital for a 3-day stay. A team conference (including Rose, Fred, Rose's physical therapist, her occupational therapist, her social worker, and her pharmacist) was called to develop her discharge care plan. The team's recommendations were forwarded to Rose's physician.

1. What do you think about the quality of Rose's health care?
2. What errors were made in this case? Can you differentiate between latent and active errors?
3. Was harm incurred? Was it likely preventable? How?

4. Identify two system failures in this case.

5. What are the responsibilities of the healthcare professionals in this case?

6. What are the responsibilities of the patient in this case? Of Rose's "caregiver"?

Discussion Questions to Launch Further Investigation

For further investigation, seek answers to these questions:

1. Two groups of patients, older adults and children, have been described as highly vulnerable. Identify others groups who are also considered highly vulnerable and explain why.

2. What is a patient advocate? What are some things that you will expect a patient advocate to do? Anticipate how you should react and participate with the advocate.

3. It is not reasonable to expect that our patients will understand the complexities of all the medical treatment they may receive. Given this, how can a patient or family member advocate for safe practices?

REFERENCES

1. The INDY Channel. Infant's Family Speaks Out Following Hospital Deaths. Available at: http://www.theindychannel.com/news/9884927/detail.html. Accessed November 14, 2008.

2. ABC News. Quaid Sues Drug Maker After Twins' Heparin Overdose. Available at: http://abcnews.go.com/print?id=3956580. Accessed November 14, 2008.

3. Los Angeles Times. Possible Medical Mix-Up for Twins. Available at: http://articles.latimes.com/2007/nov/21/local/me-twins21. Accessed November 14, 2008.

4. CNN. Second Twin Dies as Hospital Probes Heparin Overdoses. Available at: http://www.cnn.com/ 2008/HEALTH/07/10/heparin/index.html. Accessed November 14, 2008.

5. Kohn LT, Corrigan JM, Donaldson MS, eds. *To Err Is Human: Building a Safer Health System.* Washington, DC: National Academy Press; 2000.

6. National Patient Safety Foundation. About the Foundation: Our Vision. Available at: http://www.npsf.org/au/. Accessed September 9, 2008.

7. *Making Health Care Safer: A Critical Analysis of Patient Safety Practices.* Evidence Report/Technology Assessment: Number 43. Rockville, MD: Agency for Healthcare Research and Quality, U.S. Department of Health and Human Services; July 20, 2001. AHRQ Publication No. 01-E-058.

8. Blendon RJ, DesRoches CM, Brodie M, et al. Views of practicing physicians and the public on medical errors. *N Engl J Med* 2002;347:1933–1940.

9. American Hospital Association. The Patient Care Partnership. Available at: http://www.aha.org/aha/issues/Communicating-With-Patients/pt-care-partnership.html. Accessed September 9, 2008.

10. Coleman E, Smith J, Raha D, et al. Posthospital medication discrepancies: prevalence and contributing factors. *Arch Intern Med* 2005;165:1842–1847.

11. Rodehaver C, Fearing D. Medication reconciliation in acute care: ensuring an accurate drug regimen on admission and discharge. *Jt Comm J Qual Patient Saf* 2005;31: 406–413.

12. Rogers G, Alper E, Brunelle D, et al. Reconciling medications at admission: safe practice recommendations and implementation strategies. *Jt Comm J Qual Patient Saf* 2006;32:37–50.

13. Bedell SE, Jabbour S, Goldberg R, et al. Discrepancies in the use of medications. *Arch Intern Med* 2000;160:2129–2134.

14. Wachter RM, Shojana KG. *Internal Bleeding: The Truth Behind America's Terrifying Epidemic of Medical Mistakes.* New York: Rugged Land; 2004.

15. Sharpe VA. Why "do no harm"? *Theor Med* 1975;18:197–215.

16. Beauchamp TL, Childress JF. *Principles of Biomedical Ethics*, 5th ed. New York: Oxford University Press; 2001.

17. Pellegrino ED. Toward a reconstruction of medical morality: the primacy of the act of profession and the fact of illness. *J Med Phil* 1979;4:32–55.

18. National Patient Safety Foundation at the AMA. Public Opinion of Patient Safety Issues: Research Findings. 1997. Available at: http://www.npsf.org/pdf/r/1997survey. pdf. Accessed November 14, 2008.

19. National Patient Safety Foundation. The Role of the Patient Advocate. 2003. Available at: http://www.npsf.org/download/PatientAdvocate.pdf. Accessed November 14, 2008.

20. Crook T, Ferris S, Bartus R, eds. *Assessment in Geriatric Psychopharmacology.* New Canaan, CT: Mark Powley; 1983, pp. 50–51.

Safety Improvement Is in Professional Practice

Ann M. Rule, Teresa M. Cochran, Amy A. Abbott,
Andjela Drincic, Barbara M. Harris, and Keli Mu

PURPOSE

The purpose of this chapter is to understand safety from the professional's point of view. Patient safety is examined from professionals' roles within the healthcare delivery system, their experiences with patients and their caregivers and with other care providers, and the structure of their practice environment.

OBJECTIVES

After completing this chapter, you will be able to:

- Explain your own discipline's scope of practice (discipline-specific skill set)
- Describe and appreciate the contributions of other professionals in interprofessional patient care
- Apprise the issues of trust between healthcare disciplines
- Discuss the advocacy role of interprofessional teams, and identify needs that are not being met
- Explain why you as a professional need effective communication skills to achieve patient safety

VIGNETTE

A 49-year-old woman was admitted to the hospital for a right femoral (above-the-knee) amputation necessitated by nonhealing decubitus ulcers. She had several chronic conditions, including a history of spastic cerebral palsy, a seizure disorder, mental retardation, chronic urinary tract infections, chronic osteomyelitis, and bilateral lower-extremity ischemia. The patient's family accompanied the patient to the hospital. The surgery was performed without complications. Standard PRN (as needed) postoperative orders for intravenous morphine were written.

The patient experienced the onset of tachycardia, tachypnea, and increased blood pressure 24 hours after surgery. These symptoms led to an evaluation by a cardiologist. The cardiologist ruled out cardiac causes and considered the possibility that the patient was in pain. Consequently, the cardiologist requested consultation for the patient from the pain management team. Although the patient was noncommunicative at the time, her family reported that she was normally talkative, was up in her wheelchair, and attended school daily. They were concerned that the nurse would not give the patient medication for pain because she was not complaining of pain. The increased heart rate, respiratory rate, and blood pressure coupled with the fact that the patient screamed out on movement led the pain management team to conclude the patient was suffering from severe, acute postoperative pain even though she was unable to verbalize this. It is expected that patients who have undergone an amputation experience severe postoperative pain and muscle spasms.

A low-dose, continuous morphine infusion was started when it was determined that the patient was unable to ask for pain medication or manage the self-administration of morphine through a patient-controlled analgesia pump. Within a short time, the patient's blood pressure and heart rate decreased. By the next day, the pain management team was able to use the Wong Faces Scale to evaluate the patient's pain, and she was able to point to the face that indicated her pain level. By the time of discharge, the patient was on oral medications and was again communicating with her family and caregivers.

The pain management team spoke with the nurse who was caring for the patient. She admitted not administering any pain medication during the 24 hours after surgery because the patient was not complaining (in spite of the fact that her lower leg had been amputated). The nurse became quite hostile when asked about the patient and her judgment concerning the patient. She expressed concerns about addiction when using opioids (such as morphine) for pain and did not believe that they should be given unless the patient was in severe pain.

THE PROFESSIONS: ROLES, SCOPES OF PRACTICE, AND EDUCATIONAL PREPARATION

Each of us is trained from the viewpoint of a core discipline and, if a health professional, a specific profession. The professions collectively have a core set of responsibilities to those they serve. These responsibilities are described explicitly in laws and regulations, as well as being understood implicitly within each profession and by the patients served. In this chapter, we first introduce the roles and scopes of practice and provide an overview of educational preparation for some common health professions to facilitate a basic understanding of each. It is through this understanding that we gain mutual respect and are better prepared to interact and engage in patient-centered care to achieve safety for our patients. Many professions are related to the provision or oversight of health care. This chapter includes information about the professions of medicine, nursing, occupational therapy, pharmacy, physical therapy, and social work.

The Profession of Medicine

Calman published in 1994 that "the purpose of medicine is to serve the community by continually improving health, health care, and quality of life for the individual and the population by health promotion, prevention of illness, treatment and care, and the effective use of resources, all within the context of a team approach."[1] The practice of medicine involves both the art and science of healing. It encompasses a range of healthcare practices evolved to maintain and restore human health by the prevention and treatment of illness. The practice of medicine uses findings from biomedical research and technology to diagnose and treat injury and disease. The usual methods of treatment include medicines, surgery, or different types of therapy. This knowledge is combined with clinical reasoning and judgment to develop a plan of care for each patient.

The practice usually takes place during a medical encounter between the patient and physician, who establish a relationship when the patient seeks a physician's help with his or her concern. Other health professionals similarly establish a relationship with a patient. The medical encounter is documented in a medical record, a legal document in all jurisdictions.

The Profession of Nursing

According to the American Nurses Association Policy Statement (2003), "nursing is the protection, promotion, and optimization of health and abilities, prevention of illness and injury, alleviation of suffering through the diagnosis and treatment of human response, and advocacy in the care of individuals, families, communities, and populations."[2] Nursing is set apart from other healthcare professions, particularly medicine, because nurses focus on the actual or potential health problems of individuals and families while focusing on the whole person. Nurses build on the knowledge of illness and disease to promote the restoration and maintenance of health in patients.

The essential core of practice for a registered nurse is to deliver holistic, patient-centered care. This is in part achieved through use of a common language and the nursing process, which unites different types of nurses working in various clinical areas. It involves assessment, diagnosis, planning, intervention, and evaluation. After an initial assessment takes place, the priority nursing diagnoses are identified and serve as the basis for the individualized plan of care that is subsequently designed. This plan is developed around a specific nursing conceptual model or theory and best practices based on evidence-based care of the patient's problems in a particular setting. Nurses and patients mutually set measurable, achievable goals (both short and long term) and implement the plan of care. Evaluation of this plan is done, and the plan is modified as needed based on the patient's response.

Nursing is the nation's largest healthcare profession, with over 2.9 million registered nurses nationally.[2] Nurses consistently rank as the most trusted profession in the country today.[2] Although nursing requires a person to have a strong science knowledge base and be skilled in a variety of technologies, it also serves to provide individuals and families comfort and counseling, education, and health promotion to facilitate healthy lifestyles, knowledge of one's illnesses, awareness of risk factors, as well as self-care while tending to human vulnerability.[3] Nurses are educated as general practitioners who are prepared to practice across multiple and often nontraditional settings. They are accountable, responsible leaders who serve as coordinators of care for the diverse populations they serve. This care occurs in a variety of settings, including in the acute-care setting (hospitals), as well as in multiple community-based settings such as long-term care facilities, nursing homes, schools, and businesses (employee health).

After successful completion of an approved nursing program (diploma, associate degree, or bachelors degree), one is eligible to sit for the licensure examination to grant registered nursing status. Nurses can also gain higher education through a master's or doctoral degree and then can practice as a clinical nurse specialist, a nurse practitioner, an educator, a researcher, or an administrator. The Doctorate of Nursing Practice, the highest level of preparation for clinical practice, is an alternative to the traditional research-focused PhD programs.

This program is a professional doctorate such as a doctor of pharmacy, physical therapy, or medicine.

The Profession of Occupational Therapy

Occupational therapy is a profession that "enables people to do the day-to-day activities that are important to them despite impairments, activity limitations, or participation restrictions or despite risks for these problems."[4, p.5] Occupational therapists, through their interventions, enable people to gain health as well as function."[5, p.252] Settings that occupational therapists practice in are as varied as the talents, abilities, and needs of the persons they serve. It is common to see occupational therapists in patients' homes, rehabilitation facilities, industrial settings, and corporate environments.

The Profession of Pharmacy

Pharmacists are responsible for "the provision of drug therapy for the purpose of achieving definite outcomes that improve a patient's quality of life. These outcomes are cure of a disease, elimination or reduction of a patient's symptomatology, arresting or slowing of a disease process, or preventing a disease or symptomatology."[6] This responsibility is known as pharmaceutical care. Pharmaceutical care involves the process through which a pharmacist cooperates with a patient and other clinicians in designing, implementing, and monitoring a therapeutic medication plan that will produce specific therapeutic outcomes for the patient. Three major functions are involved: identifying potential and actual drug-related problems, resolving actual drug-related problems, and preventing drug-related problems.

Pharmaceutical care is intended to be integrated with other elements of health care and should be provided for the direct benefit of the patient. The pharmacist is responsible directly to the patient for the quality of that care. The fundamental relationship in pharmaceutical care is a mutually beneficial exchange in which the patient grants authority to the provider and the provider gives competence and commitment (accepts responsibility) to the patient. The fundamental goals, processes, and relationships of pharmaceutical care exist regardless of practice setting.[6]

Currently, all schools of pharmacy offer the entry-level Doctor of Pharmacy curriculum (PharmD). Although this requirement remains somewhat controversial within the profession, pharmacists are graduating with advanced degrees and are striving for more clinical roles in practice. Many go on to complete general pharmacy practice residencies, specialized residencies, and fellowships after completion of the Doctorate in Pharmacy.

The Profession of Physical Therapy

The American Physical Therapy Association's *Guide to Physical Therapist Practice* defines physical therapy's focus as restoring, maintaining, and promoting optimal physical function and quality of life related to movement and health. Physical therapists are also instrumental in preventing the "onset, symptoms and progression of impairments, functional limitations and disabilities resulting from injury, disease or other causes."[7] Settings in which physical therapists practice vary widely, including hospital, school system, corporate, athletic, rehabilitation, and industrial and patient home environments. Major changes have occurred in physical therapy education over the past several years. Direct access to physical therapy services without physician referral is permitted in 44 states and the District of Columbia.[8] To support physical therapy practice in the direct access model, minimal education requirements have evolved from post-baccalaureate certification to baccalaureate, master's, and doctoral degree credentials. The American Physical Therapy Association's Vision 2020 statement recommends that all physical therapy education programs offer only the clinical Doctor of Physical Therapy degree as the recognized credential of choice in the near future.[9]

The Profession of Social Work

Social work practice in health care is described as assisting individuals, their families, and significant others to function when illness, disease, or disability results in changes in their physical state, mental state, or social roles; to prevent social and emotional problems from interfering with physical and mental health or needed treatment; and to identify gaps in community services and to work with community-based agencies and institutions to expand the capacity of the community to provide adequate supports.[10] The National Association of Social Workers reports that half a million social workers practice in the United States, but social work is still one of the most misunderstood and often misrepresented professions. Of the healthcare disciplines, it may be the profession with the most ambiguity, even though the American Hospital Association mandates a social service unit in a hospital to meet the requirements. Social workers practice in the areas of discharge planning, hospice, oncology, public health, nursing home, and long-term care. Social workers frequently practice in settings where the primary function of the agency is social work. According to

Zastrow, "Healthcare is a secondary setting for social work. In such a setting, social workers generally function as members of a team and they need to learn to work with those in charge. Medical treatment teams are increasingly dependent on social workers to attend to socio-psychological factors that are either contributing causes of illness or side effects of a medical condition that must be dealt with to facilitate recovery."[11] In 2006, healthcare and social assistance accounted for 5 of 10 social work jobs. An additional 3 of 10 social workers were employed by state and local government agencies, primarily in departments of health and human services.[12]

PATIENT SAFETY ADDRESSED IN PROFESSIONAL CODES AND PROFESSION-SPECIFIC LITERATURE

All health professions hold high standards and use codes of ethics to describe these standards through commitments to society and those we serve. The areas within the disciplinary codes of ethics and the prominence of patient safety work in the disciplinary literature are introduced in this section.

The code of ethics for medicine is described in the American Medical Association's Principles of Medical Ethics. Key principles that support the responsibility to patient safety include I, II, and IV. These principles state the following:

- A physician shall be dedicated to providing competent medical care, with compassion and respect for human dignity and rights.
- A physician shall uphold the standards of professionalism, be honest in all professional interactions, and strive to report physicians deficient in character or competence or engaging in fraud or deception to appropriate entities.
- A physician shall respect the rights of patients, colleagues, and other health professionals and shall safeguard patient confidences and privacy within the constraints of the law.[13]

The code of ethics for nursing has nine provisions that describe the principles governing this code. Provision 8 addresses both the health needs and concerns and the nurses' responsibilities to the public. The first two statements within this provision specifically address safety. The first says that "the nursing profession is committed to promoting the health, welfare and safety of all people." The second says that "nurses, individually and collectively, have a responsibility to be knowledgeable about the health status of the community and existing threats to health and safety."[14]

Occupational therapists have a code that emphasizes providing health care to patients who are in need. The Occupational Therapy Code of Ethics states that "occupational therapy personnel shall take reasonable precautions to avoid imposing or inflicting harm upon the recipient of services or to his or her property (nonmaleficence)" and "occupational therapy personnel shall achieve and continually maintain high standards of competence (duties)."[15, p.614] In comparison with other healthcare professions, literature on patient safety and practice errors in occupational therapy is quite scarce. Although anecdotal reports, textbook cases, malpractice documentation, and regulatory board records show that occupational therapists do make errors and cause harm to patients,[16–18] systematic research on patient safety issues was not initiated until recently.[19] Systematic research is warranted to examine occupational therapy practice errors and develop preventive strategies to reduce errors and improve patient safety.

Pharmacists have long been involved in "patient safety." The culture of pharmacists is to provide "safe and efficacious" medication therapy. Much has been written about medication errors and the role of the pharmacist in preventing medication errors. The role of the pharmacist extends beyond dispensing medication, however; in fact, the pharmacist's role extends beyond dispensing the right medication at the right time in the right dose and past the administration to the patient taking the right medication at the right time in the right dose. The code of ethics for pharmacists emphasizes the covenantal relationship between the patient and pharmacist, the obligation of the pharmacist to maintain professional competency, and the importance of acting with honesty and integrity in professional relationships. Several pharmacy professional associations facilitate professional advancement of high-quality practice standards and continuing education. The American Society of Health-System Pharmacists offers a patient safety resource center on their website.[20] The American Pharmacist's Association has a significant focus on medication and medical errors. Many of their educational sessions focus on medication errors. In addition, the Institute for Safe Medication Practices was founded by a pharmacist and his nurse wife from Pennsylvania. The Institute for Safe Medication Practices website offers tips on medication safety, high risk medications, and strategies to overcome medication errors.[21]

The Physical Therapy Code of Ethics directly refers to the term *safety* as related to environmental and equipment issues, but also emphasizes the responsibility of the physical therapist in maintaining professional competence, exercising sound judgment, and protecting society from "unethical, incompetent, and illegal acts."[22] Consistent with other rehabilitation professions, a relative paucity of literature is available related to safety in the physical therapy literature base. The past decade of safety research in physical therapy has focused on understanding the nature of errors committed by novice versus expert clinicians and improvement of diagnostic skill.[23–26] In seminal work by Deusinger, physical therapists were studied to identify the types of the nature and consequences of practice errors. A taxonomy was developed that identified the dimensions of "action, error, and consequence" in physical therapy patient management. Action-type elements relate to decision making, interpersonal communication, technical or psychomotor skills, and cognitive factors related to knowledge. Error-type elements may be directly committed or may occur as acts of omission by practitioners, whereas consequence-type elements are characterized as actual, potential, social, or physical.[27] The most frequently occurring errors were associated with misdiagnosis, intervention planning, documentation, gait training, application of thermal or electrical modalities, and delegation of responsibilities to physical therapist assistants or physical therapy aides. Consequences of practice errors in physical therapy ranged from relatively minor concerns such as bruising or lacerations to more serious situations in which a preventable condition was not avoided or fracture or patient death occurred.[27] Although the latter results were infrequent, inquiry into physical therapy practice errors and understanding of the role of physical therapy in promoting safe patient care is certainly warranted.

The profession of social work has evolved with the cornerstone of practice as laid out in the Code of Ethics focusing on empowering people to enhance their own well-being.[10] This document provides a customary protocol for the practice of social work in health care recognized by the National Association of Social Workers. While providing a broad set of standards for practice in health settings, it does not address specific issues of patient safety. The National Association of Social Workers document also delineates a standard for working in interdisciplinary teams by calling on social workers to understand the functions of other disciplines and to help clearly delineate the roles of team members.

PATIENT SAFETY AND INTERPROFESSIONAL COLLABORATION

Interprofessional collaboration has been identified by almost all professions as a key aspect to improving patient safety. One of the more recent issues in safety has been the safe transition of care when the patient moves from one care location, such as a hospital, to another care location, such as a nursing home or the patient's own home. The National Transitions of Care Coalition brought together 27 different disciplinary stake holders to address the risks patients face as they transition from levels of care.[28] Transitions in care include a patient moving from primary care to specialty physicians; within the hospital, it would include patients moving from the emergency department to other departments, such as surgery or intensive care or when patients are discharged from the hospital and go home, into an assisted living arrangement or into a skilled nursing facility.[29] Breakdowns in communication among professionals particularly in making referrals and following up on the referrals made increased risk for patients. In April 2008, the coalition released tools to improve patient safety while transitioning from levels of care. Of particular interest is the coalition's recommendation for increased use of case management and professional care coordination.

Varying Definitions of Collaboration

In health care, we often speak of collaborations between healthcare professions as a patient care team. Three different team models exist for providing healthcare services to patients who are in need: multiprofessional, interprofessional, and transprofessional. In spite of the similarities among them, it is imperative to point out the differences between the three team models. A multiprofessional team is at the lowest level of the evolution scale of the team model and is often referred to as a profession-referenced model. In the multiprofessional model, professionals from different professions function more or less independently in providing care to patients. The cooperation among professionals is fairly limited, and services to the patients can be fragmented, isolated, duplicated, or even conflicting. The interprofessional approach denotes a deeper level of cooperation whereby professionals plan and evaluate services to patients jointly. Professionals from different professions pool their knowledge and skills in an interdependent manner to plan, develop and evaluate services to maximize the benefits of services to the patients. The provision of services, however, remains profession independent. This higher level of cooperation requires "members of the team to have an underlying respect and value of what each discipline brings to the care of the patient. There is a high level of trust among the disciplines along with a solid understanding of the individual discipline's scope of practice."[30, p.339]

The transprofessional team model is highest on the evolution scale of team models and requires a much deeper cooperation and collaboration among team members. Within the transprofessional approach, team members share or transfer information and skills across traditional profession boundaries and provide indirect services to the individuals who are underserved. One or two team members serve as the primary facilitators or team leaders of services and the other team members serve as consultants.

The interprofessional team model has been advocated for over 2 decades for delivering patient care services. Outcomes of interprofessional health care have been well articulated in healthcare literature, and documented outcomes include enhanced quality of care, improved patient outcomes, maximizing available resources, and provision of more holistic care.

CONCEPT OF THE "TEAM" IN SAFE PRACTICE

The literature is replete with data describing the need for health science professionals to collaborate as a team because of the correlation to increased successful patient outcomes.[31] Additionally, authors report increased job satisfaction and lower burnout when they work in interprofessional teams.[32–34]

Although the merits of interprofessional healthcare are well documented in healthcare literature, barriers do exist that hinder implementation of interprofessional healthcare services. Previous literature has suggested that noticeable obstacles consist of professionals' limited understanding of the scope of practice of other professionals, limited understanding of the significance of collaboration among professionals in improving quality of care, a lack of adequate training on the complexities and contributions of varied healthcare professionals, poor preparation of interprofessional skills, and the tendency of preserving traditional role concepts and maintaining territoriality concerns. In order to enhance the function of a collaborative interprofessional healthcare team, the terminology related to "team" must first be considered. Payne defines the term "team" as a "group of interdependent individuals who have complementary skills and are committed to a shared, meaningful purpose and specific goals."[35, p.99] In the study of organizational behavior, a critical difference between the concepts of "group" and "team" sometimes remains unconsidered in the implementation of interprofessional care roles. Robbins[36] asserts that groups exist when individuals interact primarily to share information and make decisions. Summation of the individual contributions produces a desired result, but there is an absence of "synergy" produced by the group interaction. In true team functioning, a central, meaningful focus (e.g., the patient's needs) transcends discipline-specific needs, and focusing on the common purpose generates positive synergy, resulting in an advanced level of performance or greater success than would have been possible working alone. The importance of this difference allows us to understand that just because individuals are brought together to work as a group, the group may not be performing at the level of a team.

At the center of the team is a functional level of trust. The dimensions of trust have been identified by Schindler and Thomas to include the characteristics of integrity, competence, consistency, loyalty, and openness.[37] It is suggested that integrity and competence are the most important because they form the substrate for all other actions or behaviors.[36] In order to develop skills to enhance team performance, Bassoff expands on the level of trust and presents the following four fundamental attitudes[38, pp.282,283]:

1. Attitude of openness and receptivity to ideas other than one's own: flexibility
2. Attitude of value and respect for other disciplines: a trusting of others
3. Attitude of interdependence and acceptance of a common goal: commitment to comprehensive patient care
4. Attitude of willingness to share and take responsibility

Based on Bassoff's philosophy, Luecht et al. suggest professional training must require the following student outcomes:

1. An appreciation of the skills, knowledge, and expertise held by each group so that healthcare professionals will respect and value one another's input in the total decision-making process of the team
2. Knowledge of the functional roles of each discipline within the team
3. The interpersonal skills necessary for practice in a multidisciplinary health team
4. The skills of group behavior they will need to function in the team[39, p.181]

To develop these attitudes and skills, it is clear that trust must be acculturated at two levels in order for the team to provide safe patient care. First, the health practitioner must have a strong understanding of his or her specific scope of practice and technical skills. This is a process that develops over time, but a firm grasp of the discipline-specific patient goals is necessary. For example, if the patient's needs are related to an inability to walk on uneven terrain to attend a social event in the downtown community center, the physical therapist must understand the patient needs primarily associated with strength, motor control, balance, and gait skills in order to function adequately. The pharmacist must understand potential pharmacological interventions that may contribute to gait disturbance. The occupational therapist must understand the importance of attending the social event to the patient, and the occupational therapist may explore compensatory equipment to ensure the patient's safety. The social worker also has to recognize the importance of maintained social function for the patient, but the social worker might focus on resources or policy issues preventing facility access for those with disabilities. All have specific goals and interventions related to the patient needs, and it is important to understand that the roles of the health practitioners may overlap in certain situations. For example, the physical therapist may decide to order a wheelchair, or the occupational therapist may decide to advocate for public transportation with a wheelchair lift so that even if the patient cannot ambulate he or she will still maintain the important social role by attending the event. It is critical that a healthcare practitioner understand his or her individual role, scope of practice, and goals related to each patient encountered.

The second level of trust relates to depth of understanding of the roles of other healthcare practitioners. When one understands the role of the occupational therapist, the social worker, or the pharmacist on the team, one is able to understand when disciplinary roles may overlap and when roles must remain very specific. The level of knowledge of other health professions allows respectful communication and the ability to trust that the patient's needs will be met by some or all of the group members involved. In the aforementioned example, a well-functioning interprofessional team would maintain a patient-centered focus to determine the priority of the patient's specific needs and to determine the available resources to meet the needs. In this case, the immediate priority might be acquisition of a wheelchair to maintain community interaction, but follow-up needs would be related to a course of physical therapy to eliminate the need for the wheelchair as strength and balance improve with intervention. The interprofessional team would determine the patient needs and interventions (with patient input) and identify the appropriate provider(s) for care. Well-functioning interprofessional teams avoid turf concerns because the central question is based on prioritized patient need in the context of trusting one's own skill level and the skill level of the other members of the healthcare team.

Several factors diminish optimal team function, including the design of the current healthcare system. The traditional medical model places the physician in the center of the decisions, rather than basing referrals on prioritized patient needs. This model can work effectively when the physician trusts the other healthcare providers and uses available resources, but each team member is accountable to earn such trust by providing and advocating for quality patient care. Miscommunication among health providers, blaming, lack of confidence, and limited assertiveness and conflict resolution strategies also contribute to less than optimal team function. According to the Institute of Medicine report, communication and team work behaviors are two major variables associated with healthcare safety.[40]

Blame of a particular individual when an error occurs can only promote a "punitive" culture and hinder the process of analyzing root causes and designing a more efficient and safer healthcare system.

In order to promote patient safety and provide quality patient care, each healthcare professional must learn to function as an essential component of an interprofessional team. In order to do this, not only must the practitioner develop specialized skills and knowledge central to the respective discipline, he or she must also develop a set of core attitudes and skills related to effective interpersonal and team function.[40] Effective communication, flexibility, and knowledge of self and others (both skills and limitations) will allow the development of competence and trust. Only when we understand our contributions and the talents of other disciplines can we understand the truly interdependent nature of the healthcare system and the ability to enhance patient care.

SUMMARY

Safe patient-centered care depends on our ability to perform within our own discipline's scope of practice (discipline-specific skills set) while understanding and appreciating the contributions of other professionals. In our work as health professionals, we must remain open to issues of trust among members of the interprofessional healthcare team and recognize our role as an advocate for patient safety in all of our collaborations. We can make great contributions by identifying patient safety needs that are not being met. This requires a dedicated commitment to effective communication with colleagues, other healthcare professionals, and the patient.

A CLOSING CASE

Read the following case and use the questions that follow to apply what you have learned in this chapter:

After graduation from pharmacy school, I accepted a staff pharmacist position at the hospital where I trained. After completing a 2-week orientation, I came to work on a Monday afternoon to work the evening shift. About an hour before the day shift crew left, the Director of Pharmacy accidentally splashed hydrochloric acid in his eyes. He came across the hall, and we immediately placed his face under the eyewash. He was taken immediately to the emergency department. Needless to say, everyone was pretty shook up about the incident. At 4:00 p.m., the day shift crew left for home, and the evening technician and I began to process the evening orders.

We received an order for a "stat" total parenteral nutrition solution (TPN). The surgeon was in the process of placing the central catheter into the patient as a route for administering the TPN, and nursing sent the order down and called requesting the TPN be compounded (prepared for administration) as soon as possible.

The evening technician went home at 7:00 p.m. I reviewed the orders, made the label, and began to compound the TPN. The TPN order included insulin, and I remembered that the only type of insulin that could be used in a TPN was regular insulin. I recall being somewhat concerned about the dose of insulin but decided not to contact the physician because, after all, he was the chief of staff and had much more experience with TPN than I did. After three more calls from nursing asking about their "stat" TPN (stat means "do it immediately"), I completed the compounding, and a nurses aide came to the pharmacy to pick it up. At the end of my shift, I closed down the pharmacy and went home. Even though it was an eventful first day on the job on my own, I felt that I had handled things well. The next morning, the Clinical Pharmacist and the Director of Pharmacy took me into an office and asked me about the TPN. Fortunately, the director had suffered only minor burns to his face from his accident. I recounted how I had compounded the TPN in detail. They asked me how much insulin I added to the TPN. I pulled a copy of the order and told them what I had done. They asked whether I had any concerns about the dose of insulin. I reported that I thought the dose was somewhat high but that I thought the patient may have been diabetic and the order came from the chief of staff. Then they told me that the physician who had written the order had done so in error. He had intended to write for heparin but had written the order for insulin instead. After the patient became diaphoretic, dizzy, and shaky, the nurse called the physician, and the error was discovered. Fortunately, the patient did not suffer any permanent harm.

1. What went wrong in this case? Can you identify each aspect of care that contributed to an error?
2. What can be learned from these specific errors?
3. Can you suggest two system changes that might keep one of these errors from occurring again?

Discussion Questions to Launch Further Investigation

For further investigation, seek answers to these questions:

1. What is the role of a profession's code of ethics in the context of patient safety?

2. What makes an interprofessional team effective in patient safety?

3. What can you do from your own professional perspective to reduce potential safety mishaps when other health professionals are also involved in the patient's care?

REFERENCES

1. Calman K. The profession of medicine. *BMJ* 1994;309:1140–1143.

2. American Nurses Association. ANA's Definition of Nursing. Available at: http://www.nursingworld.org/MainMenuCategories/CertificationandAccreditation/AboutNursing.aspx. Accessed November 21, 2008.

3. American Association of Colleges of Nursing, Your Nursing Career: A Look at the Facts. Available at: http://www.aacn.nche.edu/Education/nurse_ed/career.html. Accessed July 1, 2009.

4. Neistadt ME, Crepeau EB. Introduction to occupational therapy. In: Neistadt ME, Crepeau EB, eds. *Willard and Spackman's Occupational Therapy*, 9th ed. Philadelphia, Pa: Lippincott-Raven; 1998, pp. 5–12.

5. Edwards DF. The effect of occupational therapy on function and well-being. In: Christiansen CH, Baum CM, eds. *Occupational Therapy: Enabling Function and Well-being*, 2nd ed. Thorofare, NJ: Slack; 1997, pp. 556–574.

6. Hepler DD, Strand LM. Opportunities and responsibilities in pharmaceutical care. *Am J Pharm Educ* 1989;53:7S–15S.

7. American Physical Therapy Association. Guide to physical therapist practice. 2nd ed. *Phys Ther* 2001;81:13–27.

8. American Physical Therapy Association. Direct Access to Physical Therapist Services. Available at: http://www.apta.org/AM/Template.cfm?Section=Home&TEMPLATE=/CM/ContentDisplay.cfm&CONTENTID=45176. Accessed November 20, 2008.

9. American Physical Therapy Association. Vision 2020. Available at: http://www. apta.org/AM/Template.cfm?Section=Vision_20201&Template=/TaggedPage/TaggePageDisplay.cfm&TPLID=285&ContentID=32061. Accessed November 20, 2008.

10. National Association of Social Workers. NASW Standards for Social Work Practice in Health Care Settings. Available at: http://www.socialworkers.org/practice/standards/NASWHealthCareStandards.pdf. Accessed November 20, 2008.

11. Zastrow C. *Introduction to Social Work and Social Welfare: Empowering People*, 9th ed. Florence, KY: Brooks/Cole; 2008.

12. U.S. Bureau of Labor Statistics. Occupational Outlook Handbook, 2008–09 Ed. Available at: http://www.bls.gov/oco/ocos060.htm. Accessed November 21, 2008.

13. American Medical Association. Code of Medical Ethics of the American Medical Association. Council on Ethical and Judicial Affairs. Current Opinions with Annotations. Chicago IL: American Medical Association; 2008.

14. American Nurses Association. Code of Ethics for Nurses With Interpretive Statements. Available at: http://nursingworld.org/ethics/code/protected_nwcoe813.htm. Accessed November 21, 2008.

15. American Occupational Therapy Association. Occupational therapy code of ethics. *Am J Occup Ther* 2000;54:614–616.

16. American Occupational Therapy Association. *Ethics Officer Report, Comparison of Occupational Therapy Insurance Claims and Ethics Complaints (1995–2000)*. Bethesda, MD: American Occupational Therapy Association; 2001.

17. National Board for Certification in Occupational Therapy-NBCOT. *Investigations Program Manager Report, NBCOT Cases (Complaints) Broken Down by State in Past 5 Years (1995–1999)*. Gaithersburg, MD: NBCOT; 2000.

18. Ranke BA, Moriarty MP. An overview of professional liability in occupational therapy. *Am J Occup Ther* 1997;51:671–680.

19. Scheirton L, Mu K, Lohman H. Occupational therapists' responses to practice errors in physical rehabilitation settings. *Am J Occup Ther* 2003;57:307–314.

20. The American Society of Health-System Pharmacists. Patient safety. Available at: http://www.ashp.org/s_ashp/cat1c.asp?CID=489&DID=531. Accessed November 21, 2008.

21. Institute for Safe Medication Practices. Medication safety tools and resources. Available at: http://ismp.org/Tools/default.asp. Accessed November 21, 2008.

22. American Physical Therapy Association. Guide to physical therapist practice. 2nd ed. *Phys Ther* 2001;81:685–692.

23. Jones MA. Clinical reasoning in manual therapy. *Phys Ther* 1992;72:875–884.

24. Michel TH. Outcome assessment in cardiac rehabilitation. *Int J Technol Assess Health Care* 1992;8:76–84.

25. Miles-Tapping C, Rennie GA. The Canadian physiotherapy quality of care project: analysis of a derailed project. *Int J Technol Assess Health Care* 1992;8:35–43.

26. Norton BJ, Strube MJ. The influence of experience with a set of simulated patients on diagnosis of simulated patients not previously diagnosed. *Phys Ther* 1998;78:375–385.

27. Deusinger SS. A vehicle for assessing and enhancing the quality of care. *Int J Technol Assess Health Care* 1992;8:62–75.

28. National Transitions of Care Coalition. Improving Transitions of Care. Available at: http://www.ntocc.org/Portals/0/PolicyPaper.pdf. Accessed November 21, 2008.

29. National Transitions of Care Coalition. About Us. Available at: http://www.ntocc.org. Accessed November 21, 2008.

30. Caramanica L, Cousino JA, Petersen S. Four elements of a successful quality program. Alignment, collaboration, evidence-based practice and excellence. *Nurs Admin Q* 2003;October–December:336–343.

31. Rice AH. Interdisciplinary collaboration in health care: education, practice, and research. *Natl Acad Pract Forum* 2000;2:59–73.

32. Malla AK, Norman RMG, McLean TS, et al. An integrated medical and psychosocial treatment program for psychotic disorders: patient characteristics and outcome. *Can J Psychiatry* 1998;43:698–705.

33. Slade M, Rosen A, Shankar R. Multidisciplinary mental health teams. *Int J Soc Psychiatry* 1995;41:180–189.

34. Groth-Marnat G, Edkins G. Professional psychologists in general health care settings: a review of the financial efficacy of direct treatment interventions. *Profess Psychol Res Pract* 1996;27:161–174.

35. Payne V. *The Team-Building Workshop*. New York: McGraw-Hill; 2001.

36. Robbins SP. *Essentials of Organizational Behavior*, 5th ed. Upper Saddle River, NJ: Prentice Hall; 1997.

37. Schindler PL, Thomas CC. The structure of interpersonal trust in the workplace. *Psychological Rep* 1993;73:563–573.

38. Bassoff BZ. Interdisciplinary education as a facet of health care policy: the impact of attitudinal research. *J Allied Health* 1983;12:280–286.
39. Luecht RM, Madsen MK, Taugher MP, Petterson BJ. Assessing professional perceptions: design and validation of an Interdisciplinary Education Perception Scale. *J Allied Health* 1990;19:181–191.
40. Kohn LT, Corrigan JM, Donaldson MS, eds. *To Err is Human: Building a Safer Health System*. A report of the Committee on Quality of Health Care in America, Institute of Medicine. Washington, DC: National Academy Press; 2000.

CHAPTER 4

Safety Improvement Is in Systems

John M. Gleason and Kimberly A. Galt

PURPOSE

Almost all the healthcare we provide is done in a system of care. Much of the science of patient safety is built on theories related to systems. The purpose of this chapter is to provide an introduction to systems and concepts of systems analysis. Issues related to design/redesign of medical systems to improve patient safety are examined. Concrete examples are provided that translate theory to everyday experiences, including examples of how systems fail and the consequences.

OBJECTIVES

After completing this chapter, you will be able to:
- Describe the manner in which process engineering can improve systems to increase patient safety
- Explain the basic framework of systems analysis
- Describe some of the problem areas in systems analysis, including common criterion errors and the treatment of incommensurable factors
- Discuss the relevance of systems analysis and decision analysis in efforts to improve patient safety
- Describe important factors in the design and redesign of medical systems

VIGNETTE

My wife was bed bound, having experienced diarrhea for 6 weeks. How did she get to this condition?

An early visit to the family doctor resulted in a diagnosis of "flu." When her condition continued to worsen, we contacted the doctor's office again and asked the nurse to check with the doctor to determine whether tests could be conducted to identify the cause of the problem. We emphasized that my wife's sister has Crohn's disease (a fact that was documented in her medical records). The nurse called back to relay the message from the doctor: "No, it is just a long-lasting case of flu. There is no need for any tests."

Over the next several weeks, I called the doctor's office on numerous occasions, and each time was reassured that my wife's condition would soon improve—it was just the flu. Instead, her condition worsened. She was unable to sit up and required assistance to walk from the bed to the bathroom. Finally, one night my wife's temperature rose above 103°F, and we went to the emergency room. She was severely dehydrated and was pumped full of fluids. The doctors in the emergency room attempted to send her home (with the suggestion that she see our family physician the next day). Having no desire to have further involvement with the family physician, we refused to leave until someone identified a potential cause for the diarrhea and offered suggestions for further testing. One of the doctors-in-training indicated that he worked with our family physician and said that he would suggest to her that tests be conducted to look for indications of Crohn's disease. The family physician called the next day, clearly miffed that we had gone to the emergency room and sought another opinion. She did, however, finally agree that we should consult a specialist. The specialist treated the diarrhea and conducted tests that led to a diagnosis of Crohn's disease.

In recent years, the health professions have begun to recognize that patient safety errors are usually not the fault of an individual; instead, they often result from the system. An individual can be the source of problems, however, in which case there may be other indicators that suggest the need for intervention to ensure patient safety. That was certainly true with our physician who, we later found, had been involved in several other instances that reflected a lack of integrity, ethics, and professionalism. In such cases, the problem again becomes a systems problem—healthcare professionals need to police their profession better in order to weed out such individuals.

Now, some other items should have raised red flags about our family physician, flags that should have alerted the profession about questionable behavior:

- In an earlier office visit (unrelated to the diarrhea case), the doctor mentioned another condition from which my wife had supposedly suffered. My wife indicated that she had never had such a condition and asked to see medical reports to determine how the erroneous information had gotten into her medical records. The doctor indicated that there were no reports; instead, this was information that my wife's OB/GYN physician allegedly had provided to the doctor in a telephone conversation. My wife knew that could not have happened; she has implicit faith in her OB/GYN physician, and he would never have made such an error. On her next OB/GYN visit, she mentioned the issue. He confirmed that there was no such information in his records. Moreover, he stated that he had never had a telephone conversation with our physician; in fact, he didn't even know her.

- Having decided to select a new family physician, I called a representative of the health plan to determine what forms had to be completed to change primary care physicians. I also indicated that I wanted the opportunity to document, on those forms, the reasons for my request. I then contacted the doctor's office, spoke to the nurse, and asked whether I could schedule a brief meeting with the doctor. When the nurse called back, she asked whether I was planning to change doctors. I confirmed that I was but that I did not want to file the formal paperwork until I had discussed the issue with the doctor. I was given an appointment several weeks in the future. Subsequently, before the appointment, I received a letter from the health plan that indicated the doctor had requested that my family be assigned a different primary care physician. Thus, the doctor preempted my request for a new physician, thereby ensuring that my complaints would not be documented in such a request. Moreover, any complaints that I subsequently would file would appear to be a response to her decision to no longer provide service to my family. I contacted a representative of the health plan, explained what had happened, and asked whether it would be productive for me to file a complaint. I was told that it would be a waste of time, in light of the fact that the doctor had requested that my family be assigned a different primary care physician.

- The physician prescribed aspirin to an older patient who was on blood thinners. In a telephone conversation, the patient questioned the recommendation, emphasized her use of blood thinners, and asked the nurse to call this to the attention of the physician. In a subsequent phone call, the patient was told that the physician was aware of the blood thinners but did, in fact, want the patient to take the prescribed aspirin. The patient later collapsed, and was taken to the emergency room for internal bleeding.

- The physician gave me a prescription for a salve to be applied inside my nostrils. The directions for the prescription stated clearly that the salve was not to be applied in the nose. A phone call to the physician's office resulted in a new prescription—for the appropriate medicine with a similar name.
- The physician was involved in an unapproved research project that violated federal guidelines related to the use of human subjects in research. When the university's research office discovered the physician's involvement, it intervened to put a stop to her involvement.

This case raises an interesting systems-related question. How could the various parts of the healthcare system (in this case, other physicians, the insurer, emergency room personnel, pharmacists, the university research office) have interacted in a better manner to improve the chance of identifying this problem physician? Clearly, such interaction was absent because the physician continues to practice and teach. Moreover, she has been promoted in both academic rank and professional responsibility.

SAFETY IN SYSTEMS

The Institute of Medicine report (IOM) *To Err is Human: Building a Better Health System*[1] estimates that there are 44,000 to 98,000 deaths per year from medical errors in hospitals alone. The magnitude of this estimate becomes evident when you compare that with the 43,000 deaths in motor vehicle accidents or the 42,000 annual deaths from breast cancer (the eighth highest cause of death in the United States). This report further estimates that between 2.9% and 3.7% of hospital admissions result in adverse events, totaling between $17 and $29 billion in costs associated with these adverse events.

Hospital patients likely represent only a fraction of the total population at risk of experiencing a medical error. This concern was amplified by consumers, 40% of whom indicated that they were very concerned about serious errors or mistakes when they received care from the doctor's office. A reported 55% of consumers are dissatisfied with the quality of health care.[2] In early 2000, the Quality Interagency Coordination Task Force, with the Agency for Healthcare Research and Quality as lead agency, published its report to the president of the United States, "Doing What Counts for Patient Safety: Federal Actions to Reduce Medical Errors and Their Impact." This report outlined a road map for action, such as identifying and learning from errors, working with providers, and using decision support systems and information technologies to reduce errors and improve care.[3]

Root causes of medication errors usually occur in systems of care delivery.[1] Consider the case of the medication use system. The first individual who is able to prevent errors in this system is the prescriber.[4] A 1992 study involving 89 community pharmacists in five states documented the frequency and type of prescriber errors in the community setting.[5] The results revealed that the pharmacists intervened in 1.9% of 33,011 new prescription orders to resolve a prescriber-related problem. Errors of omission, commission, and interaction accounted for 60.5% of these prescriber-related problems. Illegibility accounted for 6.4% of the errors identified. Expert evaluators concluded that 28.3% of the prescribing problems identified during the study could have caused patient harm if the pharmacist had not intervened to correct the problem. Legibility of prescriptions is a widely recognized cause of medication errors.[6–10] An inability to read correctly a medication name, dose, or regimen has resulted in injuries and death. The issue is of such importance that the American Medical Association (AMA) studied the legal implications of poor legibility of medication orders. The AMA publicly reported that misinterpretation of physician prescriptions was the second most prevalent and expensive malpractice claim listed on 90,000 malpractice claims filed over a 7-year period.[11]

The IOM has identified that professional practice consistent with current medical knowledge is an essential element in achieving safety and quality in health care.[1] Reliance on imperfect memory for medical information can lead to compromised patient safety and increased rates of medical errors.[12] Both the complexity of healthcare and the lack of adequate information lead humans to make multiple errors every day. Rates of error in knowledge-based processes are also known to be higher than those associated with automatic mental processing.[12]

Automated information and decision support systems have been shown to be effective in reducing certain errors, including those associated with drug knowledge and dissemination.[13] In the case of medication prescribing, these types of errors have been shown to be reduced at the point of the prescriber through technologies.[11,14] Many respected, credible information sources are now available as electronic media on these devices. The complexity of health care requires the availability of systems to assist providers in making the best possible clinical decisions. Future trends are clearly to move all expert published information resources to electronic media.[15]

Understanding how to use our knowledge of errors to improve systems is essential to improving safety. As our understanding of the science of errors has further developed, we have come to know that in general the same error will be constantly repeated. By finding an individual to blame, we will not change this fact and only facilitate not paying attention to the important aspects of the system within which the error occurs. To prevent errors from reoccurring requires a systems approach. This is based on the knowledge that we must modify the conditions that contribute to errors in the first place.

Human Factors and the Theory of Error

The science that informs us in this area is known as human factors, attributed to the organizational psychologist James Reason.[16] Human factors is a discipline of study about the interaction of people and equipment and the variables that affect the outcome of this interaction. The discipline of human factors is built on the understanding that successful performance of the individual person within large systems depends on a wide range, in scope and depth, of complex, interdependent forces. These forces must be understood sufficiently and considered in the process of interest; otherwise, the likelihood of errors in the form of near misses or accidents and unfortunate outcomes is much higher. High-risk industries (e.g., nuclear power, aviation, transportation) have incorporated human factors engineering into their operations.

James Reason's Human Error Model is termed the "Swiss Cheese" Error Model (Figure 4–1).[16] In the illustration, the slices of cheese represent defenses built into

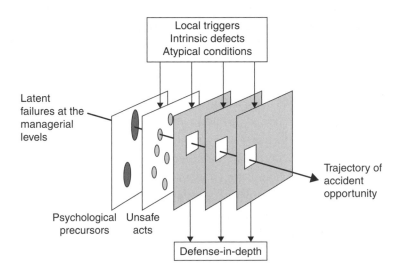

FIGURE 4–1 Human Error Model

Reproduced from Reason, J. *Human Error.* New York, NY: Cambridge University Press; 1990, p. 208. Courtesy of Cambridge University Press.

safety critical systems to deflect or stop an error; however, in reality, no system or human within the system is perfect. Imagine the slices of cheese rotating like disks around a horizontal axis. Further imagine that the "holes" in the defenses are not only repositioned because of disk/slice rotation, but are also constantly moving around on each piece of cheese and are opening and closing. In this model, when holes in the defenses line up, the error (arrow) can penetrate the defenses. This is when an accident occurs.

Through systematic research and testing, human factors engineers can also gain a thorough understanding of the likely experiences surrounding the use of equipment in development. What is the "mental workload" required—the amount of thinking and concentration exerted while using the equipment or device? The process of collecting and refining this data helps engineers design usable, effective, and safe systems.

Mental Functioning and Errors

Cognitive psychologists and human factors specialists have found that there are two modes of mental functioning: automatic and problem solving. In the automatic mode, we really do not have to "think" (i.e., our actions are unconscious and require our attention only if there is a change). Human beings are able to carry a vast array of mental models that are expert and fine-tuned processes for some minute recurrent aspects of our world. After we have a task "down," it becomes a part of automatic mode thinking. The problem-solving mode, on the other hand, requires us to gather information and compare it to stored knowledge or apply some decision rule in order to know how to act. As a result, problem-solving processes are slower. We do this in sequence and have greater difficulty maintaining our concentration and sustaining this.

The errors that occur when we are functioning in these two mental modes are also different. When we are functioning in automatic mode, our errors are called "slips," in that they usually result from distractions or failure to pay attention at critical moments. An example of an error in automatic mode would be walking into a room only to discover that you cannot remember what you came in to do.

Errors that occur when we are functioning in problem-solving mode are thought of as "mistakes." These are rules-based errors that might occur when the wrong rule is chosen, either because we have misperceived the situation or perhaps because we just misapplied a rule. Errors can also arise when we have gaps in our knowledge base, especially when we are confronted with an unfamiliar situation for which we have no programmed solution. Other factors that affect our functioning in problem-solving mode are pattern matching, biased memory, the availability heuristic, confirmation bias, and overconfidence. Pattern matching is the tendency to find patterns in situations so that we can apply previously thought out solutions. This is useful to us as learners so that we can use our prior learning in less familiar situations; however, this is also what causes us to have a patterned response. Sometimes this response is not optimal, and a resultant error occurs.

Biased memory is the tendency to overgeneralize because familiar patterns are assumed to have universal applicability. The availability heuristic is the tendency to use the first information that comes to mind. Confirmation bias is the tendency to look for evidence that supports early working hypotheses and ignore new information that contradicts it, and overconfidence is the tendency to believe in the validity of the chosen course of action and to favor evidence that supports it.[14] All of these factors affect our problem-solving ability.

Human Factors and Healthcare

The U.S. Food and Drug Administration's (FDA) Center for Devices and Radiological Health recognizes the need for human factors knowledge in the healthcare industry. This regulatory group estimates that one third of the incident reports it receives annually involve medical equipment "use error," a term referring to flawed design—inattention to human factors—rather than faulty equipment or incompetent operators.[17] Acknowledging the problem, device manufacturers have begun incorporating human factors engineering into product design. For example, enhancements in methods of drug administration, some widespread and some in use by early adopters, show great promise in reducing medication errors.[18,19]

- In anesthesia, it used to be possible for the canisters of nitrous oxide (laughing gas) and oxygen to be switched. Now the tubing of one cannot be attached to the opening or "connector" of the other. A simple product design change makes it impossible for the connections between an oxygen tank and a nitrous oxide–labeled valve to be made.
- Medication systems using bar codes, pioneered by the Veterans Health Administration and recently endorsed by the U.S. FDA, offer built-in protections that greatly reduce the risk of patients being given the wrong drug. The basic process is this: A hospital's pharmacy labels all bottles and containers with bar codes, and patients' wristbands are also imprinted with a code showing what medicines they should get. The nurse uses a handheld scanner to verify a match between patient and drug, enhancing the likelihood of accurate doses and timing of medications delivered.

- "Smart" infusion pumps for medications delivered intravenously store relevant information electronically on hundreds of drugs, including standard concentrations and acceptable dosing ranges. When a nurse programs a dose into the pump, the pump sounds a warning and gives a visual readout if the rate requested is inappropriate or outside institutional limits. If necessary, the infusion is automatically prevented.

Technology: Assessment, Evaluation, Education

The first line of defense regarding patient safety with respect to medical technology is the FDA. More than 8,000 *new* medical devices are introduced into the healthcare system annually. Only a small percentage of these devices (those classified as high risk) are required to obtain FDA approval as "safe and effective"; fewer than 80 devices receive such approval annually. Low-risk devices (more than 4,000 annually) do not require FDA approval, and only a small number (fewer than 300) of the medium-risk devices (approximately 3,500) require clinical data for FDA approval.[20] Thus, only a small minority of the medical devices introduced into the market annually require the submission of scientific clinical data to obtain FDA approval.

This suggests that patient safety with respect to medical technologies depends heavily on surveillance by the medical practitioner *after* the technologies have been introduced into the market. Feigal, Gardner, and McClellan[20] identify several ways in which such surveillance can improve safety and effectiveness:

- Detecting low-probability events that were not reported in premarket studies
- Identifying changes in risk that result from design or manufacturing revisions or modifications
- Assessing risks and benefits over extended periods or in high-risk populations
- Identifying human factors problems related to the use of the technology
- Detecting interference between new and existing technologies

Apart from the limitations of the FDA approval process, another safety risk exists with these technologies. After a technology has been approved as "safe and effective," the manufacturer or other health professionals sometimes encourage its use in the diagnosis or treatment of various other ailments; however, health insurers typically require cost-effectiveness studies to justify the use of the technology for any application other than that for which it was initially approved. This leads to efforts to assess and evaluate the use of the technology in those other environments.

Unfortunately, the practitioner cannot always rely on published reports of technology assessment and evaluation because of quality-control problems in another part of the healthcare system: the medical research literature. The importance of quality control to those at the leading edge of the medical specialties, those involved in research and the dissemination of research, cannot be understated. Practitioners dealing with time constraints in patient treatment, attempting to remain current in fast-changing fields, and guarding against interference by insurers and trial lawyers *should* be able to rely on information in journals related to their fields.

All too often, however, practitioners are obligated to second guess the quality of the reported research. During the last 3 decades, the increasing ability to acquire raw data has been accompanied by concomitant advances in computer technology that permit statistical calculations to be completed with increased ease by those who do not understand the underlying assumptions of the statistical models. This contributes to an environment in which erroneous results of medical research have a greater probability of being published. In many instances, the erroneous results arise, not from the medical aspects of the research, but from inaccurate application of decision sciences.

Two major factors contribute to errors in the research literature: improper experimental design and reporting and improper statistical analysis. These problems began to receive increased recognition during the 1980s with the advances in desktop computer technology.[21–25] Specific examples of errors in technology assessment and evaluation are discussed in Chapter 10. It should be recognized, however, that such errors need not result from complicated issues related to experimental design and statistical analysis. Instead, they may be derived from something as simple as the use of a flawed computer random number generator in the implementation of a technology assessment research protocol. Accordingly, in some instances, it may be important to first evaluate the computer technologies that are to be used in the assessment and evaluation of the medical technology.[26]

The patient-safety implications of erroneous literature are multifaceted: They impact practitioners, healthcare cost-containment, and medical malpractice.[25] Because practitioners often rely on the research literature in planning their treatment of patients, the publication of erroneous material may lead to inappropriate recommendations of ineffective or dangerous treatment or to the use of inappropriate technology in the treatment process. Not only are patients placed at risk, but the skepticism this breeds on the part of practitioners may subsequently delay their acceptance of valid research regarding related technologies or treatments.

Healthcare cost-containment is an important economic and ethical concern. The implementation of unsafe or ineffective medical procedures or the use of inappropriate technologies by practitioners, based on their perceptions that the medical research literature has shown the procedures or technologies to be safe and effective, can be expected to result in unjustified increases in healthcare costs.

Also, the issue of medical malpractice exists. If a malpractice lawsuit were to be filed relative to harmful treatment based on erroneous literature, who is *truly* responsible for the malpractice? Certainly, the researchers who reported the erroneous results, the journal that published the results, the journal referees who failed to recognize the errors, and the journal editor who selected the referees bear primary responsibility for the harmful treatment; however, the practitioner who provided the treatment, that is, the practitioner who is the proximate cause of the harm, can be expected to be the defendant in the lawsuit.

Thus, in such a case, the practitioner who attempts to provide leading-edge treatment to patients may be at greater risk of a malpractice claim than the one who relies on older treatment procedures. Regardless, it is the patient who suffers harm, but the harm is a direct result of a failure in a part of the healthcare system with which the patient has no contact. Again, the bad outcome is a system failure, but the individual on whom the responsibility is placed is the practitioner who provides the treatment. Reason[16] and Leape[13] refer to this type of error as a *latent error*, the root cause of which has existed in the system for some time (in this case, the root cause is the erroneous literature). Leape noted that the individual who is the proximate cause of the actual error has been "set up" to fail by the system.[13]

The problems related to erroneous research literature underlie several of the shortcomings identified with health professions education in a recent National Academy of Sciences report[27]:

- "Clinicians are confronted with a rapidly expanding evidence base . . . but are not consistently schooled in how to search and evaluate this evidence base and apply it to practice."
- "Students and health professionals have few opportunities to avail themselves of coursework and other educational interventions that would aid them in analyzing the root causes of errors and other quality problems in designing systemwide fixes."
- "Clinicians . . . often are not provided a basic foundation in informatics."

Accordingly, until appropriate changes are made in the healthcare education system, the onus is on practitioners to make explicit efforts to familiarize themselves with the decision sciences/medical informatics concepts necessary to evaluate the literature in order to ensure that they will not put patients at risk by basing treatment decisions on erroneous literature.

SYSTEMS

We have all been exposed to various types of systems, including systems of equations, ecological systems, and medical systems. A factor common to such systems is that if one element in the system is changed, the change often results in changes in other parts of the system. For example, if the value of one variable in a system of equations is changed, then the values of other variables change; that is, the system adjusts for the initial alteration. Similarly, we would expect a change in a medical system to result in a change in other parts of the system. Unfortunately, it is not always easy to determine how a system will adjust to a change. Considerable attention began to be devoted to this issue in the 1950s, leading ultimately to the development of the field of systems analysis and the publication of seminal books in the field.[28,29]

The various systems analysis approaches (such as cost–benefit analysis, cost-effectiveness analysis, and risk–benefit analysis) provide structured frameworks for the development and redesign of systems and decisions related thereto. Accordingly, the fields of systems analysis and decision analysis are strongly related; therefore, we consider them in a single context herein.

In this section, we first provide a brief overview of the general framework of systems analysis. Next, we consider two of the major areas of concern in the practice of systems analysis: avoiding criterion errors and dealing with incommensurable factors. Then we examine issues related to the design and redesign of medical systems to improve patient safety. Finally, we consider examples of criterion errors and improper decision analysis in technology assessment and evaluation.

Overview of the Systems Analysis Framework

In systems analysis, as with any type of analysis, we must first identify our *goals* or *objectives*; we need to define precisely what we want to achieve. Next, we must recognize that a system encompasses other systems. These other systems are subsystems of the system of interest. Similarly, the system of interest is itself a subsystem of a larger system. Accordingly, we must define the scope of our analysis; we must determine the boundaries of the system of interest (the system that is the focus of analysis in our attempt to achieve our goals). Having done so, we need to identify various ways by which the goals can be obtained within the system of interest; these various paths to goal achievement are the *alternatives*.

In order to determine which characteristics of alternatives are of interest relative to goal achievement, we define measures that will permit us to rank the alternatives relative to the achievement of our goals; these measures are the criteria. Accordingly, criteria may be viewed as measures of goal achievement. We need to evaluate the criteria-dictated characteristics associated with each of the alternatives; therefore, we develop and analyze information relative to the criteria for each alternative, and we use that information to determine our preference for one alternative versus another, using whatever decision framework is appropriate for our problem. We then implement our chosen alternative and monitor system performance in order to ensure that the system is operating as expected, making adjustments to the system as necessary.

Some Common Problems in Systems Analysis

Because the criteria drive our analysis, if we specify erroneous criteria (i.e., criteria that are not appropriate measures of goal achievement), our analysis is doomed from the outset. Accordingly, considerable research effort has been devoted to the issue of appropriate criteria and to identifying common types of criterion errors.

Criterion Errors

We consider two common criterion errors herein: attempting to maximize gain while simultaneously minimizing cost and ignoring the absolute size of the gain (see McKean[28] and Hitch and McKean[29] for a more detailed discussion of these and other common criterion errors).

Maximum gain approaches infinity, whereas minimum cost is zero. If we attempt to choose the alternative that simultaneously maximizes gain and minimizes cost, we will find that there is no such alternative. That is, there is no alternative that will achieve our goal because our measure of goal achievement (the criterion of maximizing gain while simultaneously minimizing cost) is invalid. Consider, for example, the purchase of a can of paint, where your choice is limited to brands B, C, and D. A can of paint B costs $14 and contains 5 gallons (640 ounces) of paint. A can of alternative C costs $8 and contains 3 gallons (384 ounces), and a can of D costs $9 and contains 4 gallons (512 ounces). The alternative that maximizes gain is alternative B (640 ounces), whereas the alternative that minimizes cost is alternative C ($8). More importantly, there is no alternative that satisfies the criterion of simultaneously maximizing gain and minimizing cost. (One could argue that another alternative, a generic paint, would do so if it were to sell for $7 and contain 320 ounces, but now we have extended our alternative set. In that case, we can consider other alternatives. One of those may cost only $6, but contain only 64 ounces of paint, and we again are faced with the conflict embodied in the invalid criterion.)

We can avoid this maximize-gain-minimize-cost criterion error by fixing one factor and optimizing over the other. Thus, we can fix our level of gain and then choose the alternative that minimizes cost for that level of gain, or we can fix our cost and choose the alternative that maximizes gain for that level of cost.

Often, when the error of the maximize-gain-minimize-cost criterion becomes apparent, an argument will be made that what the paint buyer really wants to do is to get the "most bang for the buck." That is, the buyer should choose the brand of paint that provides the most paint per dollar. Paint B provides 45.7 ounces per dollar, paint C yields 48 ounces per dollar, and paint D offers 56.9 ounces per dollar; therefore, choose paint D. This most-bang-for-the-buck type of criterion is also an invalid criterion. It exemplifies another common type of criterion error: ignoring the absolute size of the gain.

The drawback of the most-bang-for-the-buck criterion is that it fails to consider the level of gain needed to achieve our goal. If we need only 350 ounces of paint to accomplish our painting project, alternative C is the best choice. If we were to use the most-bang-for-the-buck alternative (D), we would pay $1 more for $512 - 350 = 162$ ounces of paint that we do not need. Thus, ratio-type criteria can be misleading. Instead, the appropriate question to ask in this case is this: Is the extra gain worth the extra cost? In this case, alternative C provides the amount of paint necessary to achieve our goal. Alternative B costs $6 more and provides $640 - 384 = 256$ more ounces of paint, and alternative D costs $1 more and yields $512 - 384 = 128$ more ounces of paint. Neither of these alternatives provides an incremental gain that justifies the incremental cost.

Criterion errors are important in practice because they often lead to "compromise" decision making. As McKean noted in his discussion of the maximizing-gain-while-simultaneously-minimizing-cost criterion error:

> If a person approaches a problem with the intention of using such a criterion, he is confused to begin with; then when he finds that it will not work, he may fasten upon any sort of constraint on gain or cost which converts this impossible test into a feasible one.[28, p.35]

Moreover, when compromise decision making occurs, it is not always possible to determine whether it was purposeful. Consider, for example, a recommendation from a study of fire-protection services conducted for a city government. The recommendation was based on the "finding" that the current configuration of fire stations did not provide "maximum coverage" with the "minimum number of stations" (attempting to maximize gain while simultaneously minimizing cost). The study team recommended that several fire stations be closed and that a number of new fire stations be constructed. They noted that the implementation of the recommendation would ensure that the city received "the same" coverage with fewer stations. Note the subtle criterion change. The erroneous maximize-gain-while-simultaneously-minimizing-cost criterion has resulted in compromise decision making that uses a different criterion (the same coverage with fewer stations) to justify the recommendation. The latter criterion is valid: Gain (coverage) has been fixed, and the criterion requires that the alternative that achieves that gain at the lowest cost (fewest stations) be chosen.

Incommensurable Factors

Determining the proper manner with which to deal with incommensurable factors—factors that cannot be measured in the same units of measurement (the apples and oranges problem)—has been one of the troublesome areas of systems analysis. For example, how do we determine the best alternative in a case in which alternative A yields 5 oranges and 27 apples and alternative B yields 12 oranges and 19 apples. This requires that we determine tradeoffs between apples and oranges, and that has been a very difficult issue with which to deal. Particularly in larger systems analyses that incorporate a variety of incommensurable factors, cognitive issues limit our ability to compare numerous alternatives on the basis of numerous incommensurable criteria.

Over the years, however, various techniques have been developed to assist in dealing with incommensurable factors. One of these techniques is the Analytic Hierarchy Process (AHP).[30,31] The AHP facilitates the decision-making process by considering the decision in the context of a hierarchy, with the goal at the top, criteria at the second level, subcriteria at lower levels, and alternatives at the lowest level of the hierarchy. The decision maker makes pair-wise comparisons of entities at each level of the hierarchy. Each entity at a particular hierarchy level is compared with each other entity at that same level, the purpose being to determine which is more important (in the case of criteria) or which is preferred (in the case of alternatives). Each pair-wise comparison of items (i.e., comparisons of the various criteria, comparisons of the various subcriteria, and comparisons of the various alternatives) is based on a nine-item verbal/numerical judgment scale, the rationale for which is based on psychological research.[32]

The pair-wise comparison process reduces the cognitive load on the decision maker, thus simplifying the decision-making process. That is, rather than having to make contemporaneous comparisons of, for example, four alternatives relative to seven criteria, the decision maker makes a series of pair-wise comparisons of alternatives. Each alternative is compared (on the nine-point scale) with each other alternative, one-at-a-time, relative to a single criterion. This process is repeated for all alternatives with respect to each criterion. Similarly, criteria are compared on a pair-wise basis with respect to the goal.

A mathematical synthesis analysis of the pair-wise comparisons subsequently determines the relative importance of each alternative and each criterion (and each subcriterion, if subcriteria are included in the analysis) with respect to its parent node in the hierarchy. Hence, the synthesis determines the overall importance of each alternative (i.e., its ranking relative to the goal), each subcriterion, and each criterion (i.e., the weight of each subcriterion or criterion) relative to the goal of the decision process. Thus, the process ultimately determines the overall priority ranking of the alternatives relative to the goal of the decision process, taking into account the importance of each criterion and subcriterion as identified by the various pair-wise comparisons.

Because the process is based on pair-wise comparisons of items at a given hierarchy level and each comparison is made without regard to the other items at a given hierarchy level, there is the potential for inconsistencies in judgments. Some inconsistency is to be expected in judgmental methods, but too much inconsistency in judgments can lead to a flawed decision. Accordingly, care must be taken to ensure that inconsistency is within acceptable bounds and to re-examine judgments that lead to unacceptable inconsistency. The AHP process incorporates methodology that recognizes unacceptable inconsistencies and that identifies judgments related to inconsistent results. Detailed discussions of the AHP are provided by Saaty,[30,31] Zahedi,[33] and Vargas.[34]

Design/Redesign of Medical Systems to Improve Patient Safety

If efforts to reduce medical accidents and errors are to be successful, they must focus on root causes—that is, errors in system design, maintenance, and operation.[13] Unfortunately, most medical systems—or nonsystems—have evolved over time with little or no conscious design effort; moreover, most were not designed to accommodate human and cognitive limitations. Accordingly, most medical systems could be significantly improved by system redesign.[13,35]

How a system should be designed/redesigned to reduce errors and improve patient safety? Leape suggests that the primary objective in this type of system design should be to make it difficult for individuals to make errors.[13] On the other hand, because of the interactive complexity of the system (discussed in

Chapter 1), it is impossible to conceive of all possible types of errors and to design the system to preclude such errors; therefore, we must recognize that errors will occur and ensure that the system incorporates buffers (design features that automatically correct for errors) and redundancies (duplications of system modules that ensure that a failure does not compromise the system).

It is also important to structure processes to reduce errors. Norman suggests a number of system design factors that are useful in that endeavor: standardization, simplification, reversibility, and the use of constraints.[36] Standardization of processes and environments reinforces pattern recognition in an attempt to reduce errors. Leape provides an example that exemplifies the need for standardization[13, p.1856]:

> There is something bizarre, and really quite inexcusable, about "code" situations in hospitals where house staff and other personnel responding to a cardiac arrest waste precious seconds searching for resuscitation equipment simply because it is kept in a different location on each patient care unit.

Simplification of tasks is useful in reducing the cognitive load on individuals as they conduct various tasks. Reversibility refers to the ability to easily reverse processes if necessary or to make it difficult to perform nonreversible processes. Constraints on processes ensure that a task cannot be accomplished until a prerequisite task is completed (e.g., a computer user not being permitted to delete a file until he or she confirms his or her intention to do so).

Finally, experience in industry has shown that the success of systems design/ redesign is highly dependent on the level of commitment by upper management. Success of similar efforts devoted to medical systems also can be expected to require analogous management commitment. Unfortunately, the increasing pressure to reduce healthcare costs can be expected to provide difficult choices for healthcare executives. In many instances (at least in the short term), they will be required to make difficult choices about increased patient safety and costly system design/redesign efforts devoted thereto.

Criterion Errors and Improper Decision Analysis in Technology Assessment and Evaluation

The management of healthcare technology requires that the integrity of the technological system (which includes the technology and the capability of the users of the technology) be routinely assessed to ensure that the system is providing accurate information. In other instances, the cost and effectiveness of technologies must be determined to justify the use of the technologies to the FDA and health insurers. We now consider cases in which assessment and evaluation studies have yielded erroneous results due to criterion errors or faulty decision analysis.

Criterion Errors

Proficiency testing of healthcare technology systems is important, not only to ensure the integrity of screening and diagnostic processes, but also for ethical and liability reasons. Although the importance of proficiency testing is well recognized, and although considerable effort is often devoted to such testing, little attention has been given to assessing the validity of the criteria used to evaluate proficiency.

The few studies that have examined the issue identified significant problems with such criteria. For example, Barnum and Gleason used systems analysis principles to examine the criteria used in drug-testing laboratory proficiency studies that were published in major medical and scientific journals from 1976 to 1996.[37] Criteria used to measure drug-testing laboratory proficiency were shown to be faulty—*thereby erroneously estimating the risks of false-positive and false-negative results*—with flawed indicators present in every study.

Three general types of criterion errors were present: ignoring the sources of false results, using an improper unit of analysis, and having improper treatment of incommensurable factors. As a result, these proficiency studies of drug-testing technology systems are of dubious value for formation of health policy about drug testing or for informing clinical decision makers about the probabilities that drug tests will correctly classify specimens.

In a subsequent analysis, the same authors found similar problems with proficiency criteria in the drug-testing laboratory certification process mandated by the U.S. Department of Health and Human Services.[37] The Department of Health and Human Services guidelines specify scientific and technical requirements for Federal agencies' workplace drug-testing programs. These guidelines also establish a certification process that applies to laboratories that perform drug testing for federal agencies.

Gleason and Barnum considered the problems inherent in the use of laboratories as the unit of analysis and identified conditions under which these problems may result in misleading conclusions, incorrect decisions, and inappropriate demands for corrective action.[38] Specifically, there are conditions under which laboratories with equal degrees of accuracy will have different false-positive reporting probabilities. Moreover, false-negative reporting probabilities may differ between laboratories, resulting in cases in which a superior-performing laboratory yields results that suggest lower proficiency than an inferior laboratory.

IMPROPER DECISION ANALYSIS IN STUDIES OF POSITRON EMISSION TOMOGRAPHY

We now consider examples of faulty decision analysis in cost-effectiveness studies published in *The Journal of Nuclear Medicine* and *Clinical Cardiology*. There are two reasons for identifying the journals herein. First, the stature of these journals indicates that errors in the medical literature are not confined to lower-tier journals. Second, when the journals received manuscripts that challenged the flawed economic analyses and provided more appropriate economic analyses, both journals immediately published the new material (one of the journals even gave it "special article status because of the important issues raised"). That is, the journals exhibited a strong commitment to ensuring that issues were aired in an appropriate manner for the scientific community.

In both cases, the original articles considered the use of an imaging technology to diagnose coronary artery disease (CAD). In one article, the technology was compared with another diagnostic technology, and in the other article, the technology was compared with results in the absence of the technology (i.e., using the technology in diagnosis versus not using it). As part of that analysis, they considered the economic impact of premature mortality from unidentified CAD. Although details are not provided herein, the following general process was employed in the economic analysis. They used the sensitivity of the diagnostic procedures to determine the number of patients with severe CAD who would yield normal results (and, therefore, would not be studied further). They then used annual mortality rates (7%) for those "missed" patients to determine 5-year death rates and used those factors in conjunction with annual lost wages to determine the loss of wages over a 5-year period because of mortality in the "missed" cases.

Unfortunately, the economic analyses were structured in such a manner as to implicitly assume that all of the deaths related to the 7% per year mortality rate occurred at the beginning of the first year. Thus, each of the deaths was assumed to incur the entire 5-year loss of wages. More specifically, the calculations implicitly assumed a 35% mortality at the beginning of the first year.

More appropriately, the effect of the annual mortality rate over the 5-year period should be evaluated by using an expected value analysis. The mortality rate should be used to determine the expected number of deaths per year, and those values should be used as weights for the potential economic loss in each year of the 5-year period to determine the expected cost over the 5-year period.

Similar errors occurred in other parts of the economic analyses in the original articles, leading to misleading results of various magnitudes. In one instance, the total cost caused by premature mortality in the absence of the technology dropped from $434,000 under the erroneous analysis to $266,000 under the expected value analysis. The articles that provided the appropriate expected value analyses also identified several other factors that should be used to further improve the accuracy of similar expected-value economic analyses.

SUMMARY

We have examined how the causes of error may be at the individual, technological, and system levels. Ultimately, however, root causes of error usually occur, affect, and are affected by systems of healthcare delivery. If efforts to reduce errors are to be successful, they must focus on root causes—that is, errors in system design, maintenance, and operation. To achieve this, such systems and the processes within these systems should be designed to make it difficult for individuals to make errors, but system complexity makes it exceedingly difficult to conceive of all possible types of errors. Thus, we must accept that errors will occur and ensure that the system incorporates buffers and redundancies to improve our opportunities to prevent these errors. The success of these system designs/redesigns is highly dependent on the level of commitment by upper management. The increasing pressure to reduce healthcare costs is a constant tension for stake holders as considerations in how to improve patient safety are brought to the forefront in our healthcare practices.

A CLOSING CASE

Read the following case, and use the questions that follow to apply what you have learned in this chapter:

A newly hired pharmacy manager was challenged to transform existing pharmacy policies to new systems as a store underwent conversion from one grocery chain to another. During those initial weeks, work was hectic, and many prescriptions were being filled for existing patients as well as for new pharmacy customers. The pharmacist, aided by a pharmacy technician, was responsible for filling these prescriptions while adjusting to the new pharmacy practices. The pharmacy technician typically filled the prescription, and the pharmacist double checked and approved the medication. They both had to sign the receipt containing the medication information confirming the dose and type. All labeled vials and storage containers were placed in a basket with the written prescription to avoid misplacing any medications. Despite these measures, the wrong medication, a narcotic schedule II–controlled substance, was given to an unsuspecting patient during that initial period of adjustment.

An unlabeled amber container with tablets sitting near the basket containing a prescription order but nothing else. It was 11:00 a.m., a busy time in the pharmacy when call-ins pour in before the lunch hour. The patient whose name was on the prescription order in the basket was waiting. The pharmacist thought the amber container had come from the basket. The technician was busy completing another job. The paperwork was already initialed, and thus, the pharmacist labeled the vial, checked the contents, and proceeded to give the prescription to the customer. Several minutes later and to their dismay, the pharmacy technician and the pharmacist both realized a mistake had been made.

In the midst of a busy time, the pharmacy technician forgot about the unlabeled container and was still working on the order the pharmacist completed and gave to the patient. The unlabeled vial contained a very similar-looking medication, but happened to be a controlled analgesic that had nothing to do with the patient's required drug therapy. Fortunately, the alarmed pharmacist was able to drive to the patient's house that afternoon and exchange the medication before the medication was taken. The patient was somewhat concerned, but actually more pleased with the reception of a gift certificate.

As a result of this incident, the pharmacist and the pharmacy technician have worked out a new system in which unlabeled vials of medicine are not to be placed on the counter of the filling area and all final signatures are not to be completed until the baskets contain the properly labeled medication. The pharmacist also carefully reviews the drug order information sheet in which a physical description of the drug is provided, including any stamped letter or symbols. She initials this description after every examination.

1. Can you identify a "slip" in this case? A "mistake"? A "latent error"?
2. The pharmacist in this case was implementing changes in pharmacy processes at the time the patient received the wrong medication. How might these system changes have contributed to the error that occurred?
3. As a result of the error that occurred, the pharmacist and pharmacy technician made design changes in the process for dispensing medication. Evaluate these changes, and describe why they may reduce errors and improve patient safety using the principles introduced in this chapter.

Discussion Questions to Launch Further Investigation

For further investigation, seek answers to these questions:

1. Develop a systems analysis framework for a system (personal or professional) in which you have an interest. Identify the goals and scope of your analysis and alternatives for achieving your goals.

2. How will you measure your preference for the various alternatives? That is, define the criteria you will use to evaluate the alternatives.

3. What data will you collect to analyze the alternatives? Where will you obtain the data?

4. Consider one of the alternatives. What are the barriers to implementation of the alternative?

REFERENCES

1. Kohn LT, Corrigan JM, Donaldson MS, eds. *To Err is Human: Building a Safer Health System.* A report of the Committee on Quality of Health Care in America, Institute of Medicine. Washington, DC: National Academy Press; 2000.

2. Kaiser Family Foundation, Agency for Healthcare Research and Quality. Americans as Health Care Consumers: Update on the Role of Quality Information. Available at: http://www.ahrq.gov/qual/kffhigh00.htm. Accessed November 24, 2008.

3. Quality Interagency Coordination Task Force. Doing What Counts for Patient Safety: Federal Actions to Reduce Medical Errors and Their Impact. Report to the President of the United States; February 2000. Available at: http://www.quic.gov/report/. Accessed November 24, 2008.

4. National Wholesale Druggists' Association. *Industry Profile and Healthcare Factbook.* Reston, VV: National Wholesale Druggists' Association; 1998.

5. Rupp MT, DeYoung M, Schondelmeyer SW. Prescribing problems and pharmacist interventions in community practice. *Med Care* 1992;30:926–940.

6. Cohen MR. *Medication Errors.* Washington, DC: American Pharmaceutical Association; 1999.

7. Feldman H. Analyzing the cost of illegible handwriting. *Hospitals* 1963;37:71.

8. Vitillo JA, Lesar TS. Preventing medication prescribing errors. *Ann Pharmacother* 1991;25:1388–1394.

9. Brodell RT, Helms SE, KrishnaRao I, Bredle DL. Prescription errors: legibility and drug name confusion. *Arch Fam Med* 1997;6:296–298.

10. Long KJ. The need for obligatory printing in medical records [letter]. *Hosp Pharm* 1991; 26:924.

11. Cabral JD. Poor physician penmanship. *JAMA* 1997;278:116–117.

12. McDonald CL. Protocol-based computer reminders and the nonperfectability of man. *N Engl J Med* 1976;295:1351–1355.

13. Leape LL. Error in medicine. *JAMA* 1994;272:1851–1857.

14. Leape LL, Bates DW, Cullen DJ, et al. Systems analysis of adverse drug events, *JAMA* 1995; 274:35–43.

15. Galt KA, Rule AM, Taylor W, Siracuse M, Bramble JD, Rich EC, Young W, Clark B, Houghton B. *The Impact of Personal Digital Assistant Devices on Medication Safety in Primary Care.* In Henriksen K, Battles JB, Marks ES, Lewin DI, editors. Advances in patient safety: from research to implementation. Vol. 3, Implementation issues. AHRQ Publication No. 05-0021-3. Rockville, MD: Agency for Health Care Research and Quality; 2005;3:247–263.

16. Reason JT. *Human Error.* Cambridge, UK: Cambridge University Press; 1990.

17. Carstensen PB. Overview of FDA's New Human Factors Plan: Implications for the Medical Device Industry. Available at: http://www.fda.gov/cdrh/humfac/hufacpbc.html. Accessed November 13, 2008.

18. Institute for Healthcare Improvement. Improving Patient Safety by Incorporating Human Factors. Available at: http://www.ihi.org/IHI/Topics/PatientSafety/Medication Systems/ImprovementStories/ImprovingPatientSafetyByIncorporatingHuman-Factors.htm. Accessed November 14, 2008.

19. Agency for Healthcare Research and Quality. Web M & M. Available at: http://www.webmm.ahrq.gov/. Accessed November 26, 2008.

20. Feigal DW, Gardner SN, McClellan M. Ensuring safe and effective medical devices. *N Engl J Med* 2003;348:191–192.

21. DerSimonian R, Charette LJ, McPeck B, Mosteller F. Reporting on methods in clinical trials. *N Engl J Med* 1982;306:1332–1337.

22. Brown CG, Kelen GD, Moser M, Moeschberger ML, Rund DA. Methodology reporting in three acute care journals: replication and reliability. *Ann Emerg Med* 1985;14:986–991.

23. Kovner C. The impact of arthritis on the quality of life [letter]. *Nurs Res* 1985;34:312.

24. Oken BS, Chiappa KH. Statistical issues concerning computerized analysis of brainwave tomography: an editorial comment. *Ann Neurol* 1986;19:493–494.

25. Gleason JM. Decision sciences aspects of medical research. *Otolaryngol Head Neck Surg* 1988;98:101–103.

26. Gleason JM. Statistical tests of the IBM-PC pseudorandom number generator. *Computer Methods Programs Biomed* 1989;30:43–46.

27. Greiner AC, Knebel, eds. *Health Professions Education: A Bridge to Quality.* Committee on the Health Professions Education Summit. Washington, DC: National Academies Press; 2003.

28. McKean R. *Efficiency in Government through Systems Analysis.* New York: Wiley; 1958.

29. Hitch C, McKean R. *Economics of Defense in the Nuclear Age.* Cambridge, MA: Harvard University Press; 1960.

30. Saaty T. *The Analytic Hierarchy Process.* New York: McGraw-Hill; 1980.

31. Saaty T. Highlights and critical points in the theory and application of the Analytic Hierarchy Process. *Eur J Oper Res* 1994;74:426–447.

32. Miller G. The magical number seven plus or minus two: some limits on our capacity for processing information. *Psychol Rev* 1956;63:81–97.

33. Zahedi, F. The Analytic Hierarchy Process: a survey of the method and its applications. *Interfaces* 1986;16:96–108.

34. Vargas L. An overview of the Analytic Hierarchy Process and its applications. *Eur J Oper Res* 1990;48:2–8.

35. Bates DW, Gawande AA. Error in medicine: what have we learned? *Ann Intern Med* 2000;132:763–767.
36. Norman DA. Stages and levels in human-machine interaction. *Int J Man-Mach Stud* 1984;21:365–375.
37. Barnum DT, Gleason JM. Analyzing proficiency criteria of health technology systems. *IEEE Trans Eng Manage* 1999;46:359–369.
38. Gleason JM, Barnum DT. A performance indicator analysis of proficiency criteria in the drug-testing-laboratory certification process of the DHHS. *RISK Health Safety Environ* 2000;11:297–307.

Safety Improvement Is Achieved Within Organizations

Bartholomew E. Clark and James D. Bramble

PURPOSE

The purpose of this chapter is to analyze, discuss, and demonstrate how safety is viewed from an organizational perspective and how organizations impact the safety of individual patients receiving care.

OBJECTIVES

After completing this chapter, you will be able to:

- Describe the differences between an individual and organizational approach to error
- Discuss how high-reliability organizations develop and maintain a culture of safety
- List and describe organizational characteristics that create an environment conducive to error
- Explain the organization's role in reducing the occurrence of medical errors
- Discuss the role of technology in contributing to error reduction
- Explain how organizations can make it easier for healthcare workers to "do the right thing"
- Explain effective organizational strategies for creating a culture of safety that intrinsically motivates healthcare workers

VIGNETTE

One afternoon, early in my career as a pharmacist, a young woman in her late 20s walked into the mass merchandiser community pharmacy where I worked. She presented a prescription for 40 ampicillin 250-mg capsules with directions to take one capsule four times daily for 10 days. Nothing was too outstanding there. Even though this episode took place during the late 1980s, before the legally mandated patient counseling and prospective drug utilization review that came with the Omnibus Budget Reconciliation Act of 1990, I was routinely counseling my patients and screening them for drug allergies.

When I asked the patient whether she had any drug allergies, she responded that she was allergic to penicillin. I realized that sometimes people who take ampicillin experience a nonallergic reaction called "ampicillin rash" or that sometimes people who have experienced an upset stomach after taking penicillin will then claim to be allergic. I asked probing questions to determine what had exactly happened in the past when she took penicillin. She stated that she developed hives all over her body and had difficulty breathing. "Hmmm . . . it was time to call the doctor and get the prescription changed to a nonpenicillin alternative," I thought. This is where the story gets really interesting.

When I called the prescribing physician's office and explained the situation, he refused to come to the phone. Instead, the person handling the doctor's phone calls returned to the line and stated in an annoyed manner that she had informed the doctor of my call and that the "doctor is aware of the patient's PEN-icillin allergy and that's why he prescribed AMP-icillin" and promptly slammed the phone down.

I then returned to the waiting patient and explained my dilemma. I could not fill the prescription as written because of my concerns about her allergy, and I informed her reluctantly that her physician had refused to talk to me about it. She then asked me whether the pharmacy across the street would fill the prescription. I explained that no pharmacist should knowingly dispense ampicillin to a patient with a penicillin allergy. She seemed unconvinced and was in a hurry to leave with a prescription to treat her urinary tract infection. I suggested that although her doctor would not talk with me that he might be willing to talk with her and suggested that she give him a call. She agreed and left the pharmacy.

About 20 minutes later, the phone rang and (surprise!) the doctor now had time to talk to (i.e., yell at) me. "Young man, if you would like to practice medicine, I suggest you go to medical school," he screamed into the phone. "Furthermore, in a medicolegal sense, if I tell you to fill it, then your [expletive] is covered." Between his rants I tried reasoning with him to no avail. I remained steadfast in my determination to not fill the prescription as written and explained that all penicillin derivatives are converted to penicilloic acid, which then acts as a hapten in eliciting the allergic response. I even tried to suggest nonpenicillin therapeutic alternatives. He remained inconsolable and hostile and then demanded my pharmacist license number so that he could report me to the state board of pharmacy. This was the end of the phone call. The patient never returned to my pharmacy, and I don't know what happened to her. End of story? Not yet.

I initiated a proactive telephone conversation with the chief inspector for the state pharmacy board that went quite well. "You let that [expletive] call me and complain about your doing what pharmacists are supposed to be doing and I'll give him a good piece of my mind. We need more pharmacists like you," he told me reassuringly. Happy ending? Not quite.

The offended physician contacted corporate management at the company where I worked, and I was almost fired by my district manager for not knowing how to maintain positive relationships with prescribers in my area. Furthermore, for about the next 6 to 8 months, our pharmacy saw no patients from either that prescriber or his two partners. They blackballed our pharmacy. Their patients transferred prescriptions out of our pharmacy to other pharmacies, and our business decreased. My reward for doing what was right for the patient and saving myself and my company a huge lawsuit was that I was ostracized and criticized by both my colleagues and management. I voluntarily left my employment at that pharmacy about a year later.

DILEMMA OF CONFLICTING PRIORITIES

This practice-based story reveals a difficult problem encountered when multiple health professionals are providing care: less than optimal interactions between professionals who are caring for the same patient. This problem was further intensified by the response of the patient care organization in which the pharmacist worked. This case illustrates the importance of both the individual professional behavior and the organizational context and framework in which the professionals are working. A key component in the provision of safe patient care is the functioning and structure of the organization within which the professional practices. In the story about the doctor who insisted that ampicillin be dispensed to a penicillin-allergic patient, aside from the less than optimal interaction between physician and pharmacist, there was also the reaction of the pharmacist's employer. The culture of that organization favored activities resulting in increased prescription sales volume. Offending a prescribing physician, even one determined to prescribe a drug to which the patient is allergic, was antithetical to the organizational goal of increased prescription sales—offend the physician, lose prescription volume. Risk management and reduction of liability exposure were not part of the equation at that interface between the professional and the the organization.

The takeaway point here is that we need to think about how professional work is carried out in organizations that may not be headed by professionals. There may not always be concordance between how professionals see their duties to their clients and how the organization's management team views professionals' duties to the organization. Consider the possibilities for role conflict—conflict between the professional role and the role of the organization employee.

Take, for example, the hypothetical chain employee pharmacist who for the past few years was following the literature on nutritional supplements and diet aids containing ephedra (before its sale was banned by the FDA in 2004) and came to the professional conclusion that he or she would recommend that consumers not use such products because of their risk profile. What if this pharmacist's employing organization had decided to boost sales of over-the-counter products by launching a promotional campaign that included setting up large displays of ephedra-based diet aids? How was the pharmacist supposed to respond when asked to promote these items actively? This example of the potential for role conflict between professional duties and organizational duties of employment is likely fairly typical.

At the organizational level of analysis, such a conflict represents a dysfunction. Organizations hire professionals for their professional expertise, knowledge, and skills. For the organization to reduce this relationship to one of just hiring the license of the professional that is legally required to perform certain duties (i.e., dispensing prescriptions to the public) is to ignore the true value that the professional brings to the organization. From a broader perspective, the organization's long-term goals and health may be best served by trusting and using fully the knowledge and expertise that professionals bring to the organization. In the previous ephedra promotional campaign example, what if the organization had first consulted with its pharmacists before launch? Sales may not have been as robust in the following quarter, but in the long term, the organization may very well have avoided civil liability for having actively promoted use of products later shown to have a track record of serious health risks.

The same dynamic can apply in situations in which employed professionals see situations with potential for error or patient harm. If they are confronted with resistance or disdain when they try to bring managerial attention to such problems, the organization misses a valuable opportunity for continuous quality improvement. Furthermore, the professional(s) involved is given the wrong message and is likely to either become frustrated and leave the organization (thus increasing costs through unnecessary recruitment and training activities) or sullenly remain without making the "mistake" of pointing out problems again. Either way, both the organization and its patients lose. It is also important to consider not only the internal dynamics of the organization where the health professional practices but also the external environment within which the organization resides. The culture of an organization can be affected by the external environment (e.g., competitive economic pressures) as well as by its internal membership. Strategic thought, rather than knee-jerk responses to immediate exigencies, is needed for organizations to respond effectively to external challenges while maintaining an internal culture of safety.

MEDICAL ERRORS FROM AN ORGANIZATIONAL PERSPECTIVE

In addition to the obvious harm that is caused to patients who experience an error, the costs associated with medical errors are staggering. In 1997, Bates et al. estimated that medical errors cost more than $5 million in a large teaching hospital.[1] Medical errors that jeopardize patient safety can and do occur at any point along the healthcare continuum and across healthcare settings, including hospitals, physicians' offices, nursing homes, pharmacies, and home health care.

Medical errors often result in adverse events. Although medical errors may not result in harm, they often do lead to an adverse event. Later in the chapter, we argue that although all medical errors do not result in an adverse event, it is vital that all errors are recognized and addressed to avoid even the possibility of an adverse event. It is important to recognize the inherent risk associated with treating patients and to recognize that some adverse events are not preventable, as the lead story in this chapter illustrates. A patient who experiences anaphylactic shock and dies after receiving an antibiotic to which there is a known allergy is an entirely preventable adverse event.

Medical errors and adverse events often result from medication errors, surgical errors, missed diagnoses, misinterpretation of medical orders, equipment failure, and organizational or system errors. Although medication, surgical, and diagnostic errors are the easiest to detect and the most visible, there is increasingly a growing consensus that medical errors are, in large part, a result of healthcare organizations having systems in place that fail to address quality and safety appropriately. Such organizational deficiencies may include the manner in which the work is carried out and resources allocated in the course of caring for patients. Indeed, Leape et al. reported that failures at the organizational or system level accounted for over 75% of adverse drug events.[2] Additionally, the allocation of resources (such as nurse staffing) influences the incidence of adverse events after major surgery.[3] This evidence has led many to believe that most of the errors are organizational or system related and not a result of individual misconduct and negligence by well-trained and well-meaning individuals who, like everyone else, can make mistakes. Efforts to reduce the rate of medical errors must focus on and require changes at the organizational and system levels and should avoid simply trying to change individual behavior.

High-Reliability Organizations and a Culture of Safety

Organizations that are considered high-reliability organizations perform successfully under very challenging conditions with very low levels of failures.[4] Healthcare professionals and institutions are called on to provide technically challenging and complex healthcare services to patients safely and efficiently. Failure to do so can result in catastrophic consequences. To what degree can healthcare organizations be considered a high-reliability organization? For comparison, we turn to the naval aviation example. It is generally accepted that naval aviation is a classic example of a high-reliability organization, as it provides continuous operations in the face of high levels of intrinsic risks with a very low rate of catastrophic failure. Gaba et al. reported a rate of 1.5 accidents per 100,000 hours flown that included a fatality or greater than $1 million in damage.[4] This rate includes both shore- and carrier-based operations and, considering the complexity and unique demands of naval operations, represents a very low rate. Data on healthcare organizations seem to indicate that the error rate is much higher than it is in naval operations.[5–7] Although there are specific differences in organizational and operational characteristics between the healthcare industry and naval aviation, the common element and key across all high-reliability organizations is the existence of a culture of safety that is not affected by the inherent risks and challenges in a changing environment.[8,9]

It is incumbent on healthcare organizations to develop the culture of safety. Healthcare organizations must (1) become preoccupied with avoiding failure (i.e., medical errors and adverse events), (2) seek out and defer to experts wherever they are found and whomever they may be, (3) learn from the occurrence of medical

errors with a willingness to adapt while avoiding the convenience of simple explanations (e.g., "it was his fault"), and (4) prioritize all activities such that safety is
the guiding principle. Incorporating these ideas is essential in developing a culture
of safety.[10] Next, three necessary components of a safety culture are described as
they apply to healthcare organizations.

Become Preoccupied with Avoiding Failure

First, there must be a preoccupation with avoiding failure. To avoid error, healthcare workers must look for errors so they can be avoided altogether or corrected before an adverse event occurs. To take effective action on medical errors,
organizations must recognize the existence of latent errors that may have delayed
consequences and thus are not seen as salient to the safety culture of the organization. Adverse events are not necessarily the result of one major oversight or catastrophic error; rather, they are the result of an accumulation of small and
sometimes unnoticed errors. Many times, healthcare workers may commit an error
but not recognize it as such. For example, a hospital worker may begin to transport the wrong patient to the radiology department and realize along the way that
they have the wrong patient, or a pharmacist may reach for and momentarily re-
trieve the wrong medication for a patient. Errors of this type can be easily corrected
before the wrong patient ever arrives at the radiology department or a patient receives the wrong drug. Because correction is easy, such events may not be seen as
errors because they were not carried through to their logical conclusions and caused
minimal disruption of patient care work flow—no harm, no foul. Such incidents,
however, should be recognized as errors in the process of care and used by the organization as opportunities for learning how to prevent potential harm to patients.
Without recognizing and addressing how such "nonevents" creep into the process
of care provision, more serious adverse events are more likely to occur.

The lack of perceived salience of the error results in smaller errors not being recognized as such. Rather, they are seen more so as disruptions of the work process.
Thus, the worker who transports the wrong patient or the pharmacist who grabs the
wrong drug may view his or her actions as mere disruptions in accomplishing the
work and not take the time to examine how the incident occurred, assess its potential harm, and evaluate means to avoid future recurrence. For example, in the case
of the pharmacist who initially selects the wrong medication from the shelf, instead
of simply putting it back and then selecting the correct medication, the pharmacist
should also assess why and how this occurred. This assessment may lead the pharmacist to decide that similarly packaged but different drugs should be stocked in

separate parts of the pharmacy to avoid this type of latent error that may result in an adverse event in the future. Organizations must welcome and encourage the recognition and reporting of such latent errors. Then the errors can be analyzed, and the organization as a whole can learn from them. Such welcoming would result in a culture that emphasizes identification of not only overt errors that cause adverse events, but also of any latent errors that occur—an important addition to any organization's continuous quality improvement program.

Seek Out and Defer to Experts

Second, it is vital to recognize expertise regardless of where or within whom it may reside. The potential for dysfunction among multiple disciplines required to treat patients requires that those with expertise most pertinent to a given patient care situation be sought out and given voice. This illustrates the important need for communication and mutual respect among those involved in the continuum of patient care. Members of the team must work together to make it easier to do the right thing for the patient. If the organization has safety as its main guiding principle, then the organizational culture must allow all healthcare team members the opportunity to speak up. The hierarchy that exists in healthcare often works to discourage open communication "up the line." For example, nurses, medical residents, or other healthcare workers may be hesitant to voice concerns about the risks they believe are present in the organization based on the latent errors they have observed. Perhaps more importantly, they must be empowered by the organizational culture to immediately prevent potential medical errors they see occurring.

A Need for Empowerment

A surgical resident clearly recalls that in a conversation with a now-anesthetized patient that the patient, the patient's spouse, the resident, and the attending surgeon had decided to perform a lumpectomy rather than a radical mastectomy; however, the patient's chart specifies a radical mastectomy. The attending surgeon really doesn't recall the conversation and wants to proceed according to what appears in the chart. The resident must be empowered to speak up and initiate activities to resolve this incongruity, including checking with the spouse or even postponing the surgery until clarification is obtained.

As those involved speak up, senior physicians and administrators must listen and take time to resolve the concerns. For the health of the organization and the safety of its patients, healthcare team members must be humble enough to listen to warnings and, conversely, not be afraid to speak truth to power.

Activities Focused on Safety

Third, all healthcare activities must be done with a focus on safety. To illustrate, consider cytotechnology laboratories that screen Pap smear slides. Misreading Pap smear slides can result in undiagnosed cervical cancers that metastasize or can result in unnecessary surgeries for cancers that were never present. To avoid these errors, cytotechnology laboratories must always operate with a focus on safety; however, as reported in a 1994 National Association of Boards of Pharmacy newsletter, testimony by the American Society for Cytotechnology before the U.S. House of Representatives Subcommittee on Government Oversight and Investigation in the late 1980s indicated otherwise.

> When profit margins are tight, lab managers look for ways to pare down or streamline the lab operation. One way to do this is to minimize or eliminate time-consuming quality control procedures that "interfere" with screening productivity. Since clinicians tend not to recognize the costs or importance of quality assurance, they tend to make a decision based on low cost and convenience. Since many cytology laboratories compete strenuously for clinician business, they must cut corners to survive. This self-fulfilling system is driven by economic factors rather than quality, and the minimization or elimination of quality control methods allows badly collected or badly diagnosed Pap smears to slip through the cracks.[11]

When work loads are too heavy or economic factors too strong, they have the power to overshadow the safety culture, and the focus on safety is compromised. Safety must be incorporated throughout the organization. This focus requires organizations to manipulate organizational characteristics integral to safety, including work flow, staffing levels, reporting relationships, and leadership characteristics, so the culture of safety prevails despite a continually changing environment.[9]

To illustrate how the three concepts of safety discussed above are intertwined, consider the real-life case, as reported by CNN (2003), in which a patient was told that she had breast cancer and subsequently underwent a double mastectomy. After the surgery, the doctors admitted that the surgery was unnecessary, that it was all a mistake, and that the patient did not have breast cancer. Applying the safety concepts discussed here, consider the following questions:

- Did the organization lack focus in areas that contributed to this error?
- What latent errors were not recognized?
- Did the organization have sufficient communication channels to help competent, well-trained, well-meaning healthcare workers avoid making an incorrect diagnosis and to avoid performing unnecessary and destructive surgery?
- Did the hierarchy or culture of the organization stifle communication?

IMPLICATIONS OF AN ORGANIZATIONAL PERSPECTIVE

Poka-yoke (po' kah yo' kay) is a Japanese term that means "prevention of error by inadvertent action." The term "to err is human" clearly implies that organizations that employ humans will encounter errors. The key, from an organizational perspective, is to design systems that make the occurrence of errors much less likely and allow for immediate recognition and response to both overt and latent errors as they occur. Such recognition includes "fixing" the underlying cause(s) of the error so that it does not recur. Under the assumption that healthcare organizations employ well-trained and well-meaning healthcare workers concerned about doing the right thing and avoiding errors, it thus becomes the organization's responsibility to (1) make it easier for workers to do the right thing and (2) make it easier for employees to recognize mistakes so that corrective measures can be taken and, if necessary, to allow the person to stop the flow of work before an adverse event occurs.[12]

Technology for Improving Safety

The application of barcoding is one example of health improvement technology (see the FDA's final rule on barcodes in the Appendix at the end of this chapter). As organizations implement technology for the purpose of improving patient safety and quality of care, they must do so cautiously so as not to introduce new, unintended, and unanticipated errors caused by a change in work procedure or work flow. New technology, or the use of technology, may increase the complexity of tasks and intrinsically increase error potential. For example, there have been cases in which a hospital used a barcode system for medication administration to patients. It then discovered that the person passing medications had copies of patient barcodes in the medication room and did all of the patient wristband scanning ahead of time before going down the hall to patients' rooms for administering medications. The whole point of having the barcode system was to prevent medication administration errors by scanning the patient wristband barcode just before administering the medication to the patient. This "work-around" might be a result of the technology "intruding" on older, less time-consuming procedures.

Thus, although the introduction of new technology is intended to make it easier for healthcare workers to do the right thing, organizations must work continuously to discover the unintended consequences that the use of the technology may produce. This process should be designed to reveal how work flow can be best designed to integrate the technological improvement so the purpose of its insertion into the process is accomplished (i.e., improved patient safety).

Making It Easier to Do the Right Thing

For organizations to make it easier for healthcare workers to do the right thing, they must examine carefully how work tasks are carried out. Then, workflow redesign can be accomplished in a manner that minimizes the possibility of error. For example, in a case published in the *Annals of Internal Medicine*, a patient recovering from surgery was apparently administered insulin rather than heparin to flush a central line, resulting in severe hypoglycemia.[13]

How might this case be used as an example to identify the organizational or systematic changes that could have helped the nurse administer the right medication? First, recognize that some place blame on the healthcare worker. After all, if the vial labels had just been read correctly in the first place, this adverse event would never have happened. Although true, we have already addressed the notion that human beings make errors, and the need for minimizing errors exists. Thus, establishment of a culture of safety requires that we need to move beyond the individual as the unit of analysis and continually examine and analyze the organizational factors that contribute to error. For example, if the drugs were located in separate areas on the floor or if the vials were distinctively different (e.g., different sizes or label colors), would this error be less likely to occur?

Recognizing Errors and Accomplishments

As mentioned previously, most adverse errors are not the result of a one-time catastrophic event. Rather, they result from a series of slips or disturbances that went unnoticed until the error became more salient. Furthermore, recognizing and correcting the cause of errors is only one side of the equation. Rewarding accomplishment can be considered a worthwhile reinforcement of correct behaviors, and taking pride in one's work is a satisfying experience; nevertheless, pride and fear are in many ways two edges of the same blade. Although Deming[14] speaks of "driving out fear" in his 14 Points for Management, we might also consider the importance of driving out pride. At first blush, this may seem counterproductive. Isn't it the goal of the organization to further the positive contributions by its employees and to instill pride in organizational membership? The answers to these questions are a guarded "Yes, but. . . ." Although it is important for healthcare workers to receive corrective feedback when mistakes are made and to receive recognition for positive contributions, avoidance of the former and seeking the latter should not be the driving forces behind their work ethic. Thus, organizations must develop a culture that allows individuals to neither fear doing the wrong thing nor engage in counterproductive competition with other organization members to do the right thing. The Institute of Medicine report suggests creating a "blame-free" working environment to encourage error reporting and consequent error reduction.[5] We maintain that such a culture must be neutral in its affect. The organization needs to maintain a balance between praise and correction so that its goal of safe, competent patient care is achieved. Recognition of error and of its prevention are ways for the organization to educate itself continually in the discovery of avenues for continuous quality improvement. Thus, overemphasis of either praise or correction may be counterproductive to the organization. This is a delicate balancing act at the interface of the healthcare worker and the organization.

Consider again the story about the penicillin-allergic patient at the beginning of this chapter. The pharmacy organization criticized the pharmacist for "offending" the prescriber while not recognizing that the pharmacist had prevented a serious adverse event. Furthermore, he had likely saved the organization from the lawsuit that most certainly would have followed if he had dispensed the ampicillin as ordered by the prescriber. In contrast, the organization should have established a culture supportive of pharmacists discovering and preventing errors—even if doing so might "offend" a prescriber. A pharmacist more driven by fear of offending prescribers or receiving criticism from their organization might relent and just say "Yes, doctor" in an obvious drug allergy situation; this would be to the detriment of all involved (patient, pharmacist, physician, and pharmacy organization). An organization with the "neutral affect" would neither name someone "employee of the month" nor nearly fire him for preventing such an error. It would, however, recognize the importance of his or her error discovery and prevention of patient harm. Furthermore, the organization would have supported his or her decision regardless of the prescriber's bruised ego. In essence, the culture of the organization should promote healthcare workers doing the right thing because it is the right thing, not because they are seeking praise or avoiding punishment.

Pride and ego were also working to the detriment of the physician in the ampicillin example. Here was a situation in which a licensed pharmacist saw fit to bring a serious error to the physician's attention—an error that the physician did not recognize as such. The prescriber's immediate impulse was to demand compliance with his original prescription as written. Here was a red flag waiving in his face, and all he could think about was "being right" instead of "doing right." His pride and hubris blinded him to the seriousness of the situation.

SUMMARY

Individuals and organizations approach error from different perspectives. High-reliability organizations are preoccupied with safety and work to develop an environment that minimizes error and makes it easier for healthcare workers to "do the right thing." They also make it easier to recognize mistakes so that corrective action can be taken. They encourage workers to stop the flow of work before an adverse event occurs. Recognition of error and its prevention are critical to an organization's efforts in continuous quality improvement.

A CLOSING CASE

Read the following case, and use the questions that follow to apply what you have learned in this chapter:

In April of 1990, I experienced an unexplained pain in my groin. The pain was so acute that I went directly from work to the emergency room (ER). The ER physician suggested that the problem was most likely a hernia, but he was not certain. He let me know that a referral to a urologist by the ER would be necessary to confirm the diagnosis. He said that I should expect a call from the urology service within a week or two. The ER initiated no additional follow-up about my progress after my visit.

In July (3 months after my ER visit), with summer vacation plans looming, I realized the urology department had not yet contacted me. During this 3-month period, the pain came and went. I quickly learned to avoid certain activities (like earning more than a "B" in my tennis class!). In mid July, I took it upon myself to call urology. By late July, I finally saw and was evaluated by a urologist, and the hernia diagnosis was quickly confirmed. The urologist indicated that the course of treatment was surgery. I went to see a surgeon. After a couple of outpatient visits for evaluation, the surgeon performed an outpatient surgical procedure to repair my hernia.

In a follow-up with the surgeon 2 or 3 weeks later, he told me that unless I experienced any additional pain or complication I was finished with this episode of care. During this visit, the surgeon could not find any record of the surgery in my chart, although he was sure he had personally operated on me and I was sure because I was still feeling the pain of recovery.

One month after my successful surgery I received a call from the urology department to schedule me for an appointment. Under the impression that my episode of care was complete, I asked why they were calling me to schedule an appointment. They quickly responded that they had received a referral from the emergency department (better late than never, I guess!).

You are the organizational consultant brought in to help resolve the situation surrounding this case. Although there was no real harm to the patient, the health system CEO is concerned that a similar scenario surrounding a malignant melanoma or other equally serious diagnosis might result in significant patient safety issues and liability for harm.

1. What error(s) occurred in this case? Describe how individual and organizational approaches to error might explain the errors that occurred. How did the organization contribute to the occurrence of error(s)?
2. How might a high-reliability organization respond to the discovery of such error?
3. List and describe likely organizational characteristics that created the environment in which the error(s) occurred.
4. How might technology have contributed to or reduced the possibility of the error(s)?
5. List strategies that the organization could implement to motivate healthcare workers to become part of a culture of safety and ultimately do the right thing.

Discussion Questions to Launch Further Investigation

For further investigation, seek answers to these questions:

1. Think about a healthcare organization for whom you have worked or volunteered. How do individuals in this organization respond to a patient safety error? How do you think the organization would respond?
2. What strategies does this organization employ to reduce errors? Do these strategies encourage error reporting and consequent error reduction?
3. What change would you recommend to improve patient safety in this organization?

REFERENCES

1. Bates DW, Spell N, Cullen DJ, et al. The costs of adverse drug events in hospitalized patients. *JAMA* 1997;227:307–311.
2. Leape LL, Brennan TA, Laird N, et al. Systems analysis of adverse drug events. *JAMA* 1995;274:35–43.
3. Kovner C, Gergen PJ. Nurse staffing levels and adverse events following surgery. *Image J Nurs Sch* 1998;30:315–321.
4. Gaba DM, Singer SJ, Bowen JD, Ciavarelli AP. Differences in safety climate between hospital personnel and naval aviators. *Hum Factors* 2003;45:173–185.
5. Kohn L, Corrigan J, Donaldson M, eds. *To Err is Human: Building a Safer Health System.* Washington DC: National Academy Press; 2000.
6. Lagasse RS. Anesthesia safety: model or myth? A review of the published literature and analysis of current original data. *Anesthesiology* 2002;97:1609–1617.
7. Leape LL, Brennan TA, Laird N, et al. The nature of adverse events in hospitalized patients: results of the Harvard Medical Practice Study II. *N Engl J Med* 1991; 324:377–384.
8. Mearns KJ, Flin R. Assessing the stage of organizational safety—culture or climate? *Curr Psychol* 1999;18:5–13.
9. Goodman GR. A fragmented patient safety concept: the structure and culture of safety management in healthcare. *Hosp Topics* 2003;81(2):22–29.
10. Frankel A, Haraden C. Shuttling toward a safety culture. *Mod Healthcare* 2004; 34(1):21.
11. National Association of Boards of Pharmacy. Pharmacist workloads and public safety. *NABP Newsletter* 1994; 23(2):9,10,16 17.
12. Barry R, Murcko AC, Brubaker CE. *The Six Sigma Book for Healthcare: Improving Outcomes by Reducing Errors.* Chicago: Health Administration Press; 2002.
13. Bates DW. Unexpected hypoglycemia in a critically ill patient. *Ann Intern Med* 2002;137:E110–E117.
14. Deming WE. *Out of Crisis.* Cambridge, MA: MIT Press; 2000.

Appendix

FDA Issues Bar Code Regulation. February 25, 2004.
Available at: http://www. fda.gov/oc/initiatives/barcode-sadr/fs-barcode.html.
Accessed December 18, 2008.
FDA Issues Bar Code Regulation
February 25, 2004

TODAY'S ACTION

In an effort to improve patient safety in the hospital setting by reducing medication errors, the Food and Drug Administration (FDA) has published a final rule titled, Bar Code Label Requirements for Human Drug Products and Biological Products.

THE FINAL RULE

The FDA is issuing a final rule that requires "bar codes" on most prescription drugs and on certain over-the-counter drugs. Bar codes are symbols consisting of horizontal lines and spaces and are commonly seen on most consumer goods. In retail settings, bar codes identify the specific product and allow software to link the product to price and other sales- and inventory-related information. FDA's bar code rule uses bar codes to address an important public health concern—medication errors associated with drug products.

HOW WOULD IT WORK?

The final rule requires linear bar codes on most prescription drugs and on over-the-counter drugs commonly used in hospitals and dispensed pursuant to an order. The bar code must, at a minimum, contain the drug's National Drug Code (NDC) number, which uniquely identifies the drug.

For blood and blood components intended for transfusion, the final rule requires the use of machine-readable information in a format approved for use by FDA. The machine-readable information must include, at a minimum, the facility identifier, the lot number relating to the donor, the product code, and the donor's ABO and Rh.

Bar codes on drugs would help prevent medication errors when used with a bar code scanning system and computerized database. This system would work as follows:

- A patient is admitted to the hospital. The hospital gives the patient a bar-coded identification bracelet to link the patient to his or her computerized medical record.
- As required by the rule, most prescription drugs and certain over-the-counter drugs would have a bar code on their labels. The bar code would reflect the drug's NDC number.
- The hospital would have bar code scanners or readers that are linked to the hospital's computer system of electronic medical records.
- Before a healthcare worker administers a drug to the patient, the healthcare worker scans the patient's bar code. This allows the computer to pull up the patient's computerized medical record.
- The healthcare worker then scans the drug(s) that the hospital pharmacy has provided to be administered to the patient. This scan informs the computer which drug is being administered.
- The computer then compares the patient's medical record to the drug(s) being administered to ensure that they match. If there is a problem, the computer sends an error message, and the healthcare worker investigates the problem.
- The problem could be one of many things:
  ○ Wrong patient
  ○ Wrong dose of drug
  ○ Wrong drug
  ○ Wrong time to administer the drug
  ○ The patient's chart has been updated and the prescribed medication has changed

So, for example, a bar code system could prevent a child from receiving an adult dosage of a drug and prevent a patient from mistakenly receiving a duplicate dose of a drug he or she had already received. A bar code system can also allow the computer to record the time that the patient receives the drug, ensuring more accurate medical records.

Improving Patient Safety

The Institute of Medicine and other expert bodies have concluded that medical errors have substantial costs in lives, injuries, and wasted healthcare resources, and that drug-related adverse events are a major component of those errors.

FDA estimates that the bar code rule, once implemented, will result in more than 500,000 fewer adverse events over the next 20 years. Thus, FDA estimates a 50% reduction in medication errors that would otherwise occur when drugs are dispensed or administered, even though some hospitals that currently have bar code systems in place report a higher error reduction from bar code usage.

OTHER BENEFITS

Patients would avoid pain, suffering, and extensions of hospital stays with an estimated value of $93 billion over the next 20 years. In addition, hospitals are expected to avoid litigation associated with preventable adverse events, reduce malpractice liability insurance premiums, and increase receipts from more accurate billing procedures.

Also, the bar coding system could help with inventory control for drug manufacturers, wholesalers, and pharmacists, as well as efficiencies in ordering and billing.

Culture of Safety in Healthcare Settings

Janet K. Graves, Pat Hoidal,
and Robert J. McQuillan

PURPOSE

The purpose of this chapter is to describe the effects of culture on safety and how a healthcare organization can develop a culture of safety.

OBJECTIVES

After completing this chapter, you will be able to:

- Explain the concept of a culture of safety
- Identify values that compete with the valuing of safety
- Describe the role of organizational leaders and individual health professionals in fostering a culture of safety
- Contrast the concepts of a blame-free culture and a just culture
- Explain how the culture of safety can be measured and compared across institutions
- Describe ways to develop a culture of safety

VIGNETTE

Susan was excited to start her first day on the job as a registered nurse. She had been through 2 weeks of orientation for the SafetyFirst Medical Center and had participated in long presentations on topics such as "our culture of safety." Now she was actually going to start caring for patients, and she would have a "preceptor" for 6 weeks to help her transition into her new role and be sure that she was a "safe" nurse. Everyone was friendly and happy to have her join the staff.

Susan was assigned to care for four patients on the medical unit, earning its name because each patient had multiple medications. Susan wrote a schedule so that she would be able to give all of the medications on time. "Don't work so hard at it," her preceptor said, "you'll make the rest of us look bad."

One of the medications Susan was supposed to give was an insulin injection. She drew up the insulin and asked her preceptor to check it, as the rule is that two RNs should check the insulin dosage. Her preceptor glanced at the syringe from a few feet away. "Yeah, that looks right," she said. "I'm sure your young eyes can see that little line better than mine. I wish we would get better syringes that you could see better, but they told us we had to use these first."

Susan went into Mr. A's room to administer his 8 a.m. medications. He did not have an armband for identification. You must be new here," he said. "Everyone knows me, and I'm not wearing that thing on my arm. It is in my table if you have to see it."

Ms. B's physician left a new order on her chart for an antibiotic. The secretary typed the forms, and the charge nurse sent it to the pharmacy along with a fax of the written order. Susan received the new medication and went to Ms. B's chart to check it. The order looked as though it said 800 mg, but everyone had signed off on 500 mg. Susan showed it to the charge nurse. "It has to be 500 mg, honey—that's what he always orders." "Maybe," Susan thought, "but this person does weigh 350 pounds, so he might have ordered more." "No, we can't interrupt Dr. M. to find out: he'd have our head—just give the 500 mg" said the charge nurse.

Susan asked her preceptor to help her get Ms. B out of bed and onto the commode. The patient was a bit unsteady, and with her large size, Susan knew it would be safer if she had help. Her preceptor called on her phone and said, "I'm too busy—I've got six lights to answer; just do the best you can."

Even though this Medical Center was named SafetyFirst, its culture was not focused on safety. Luckily, this is a made-up situation, and thus, we can create a happy ending. Because Susan had taken an intraprofessional class on safety last year, she knew just what to do. What would you do?

THE CONCEPT OF CULTURE

The term "culture" refers to beliefs, attitudes, and values that are shared within a group of people.[1] Edgar Schein defined culture as "a pattern of shared basic assumptions that a group has learned as it solved its problems of external adaptation and internal integration, that has worked well enough to be considered valid and, therefore, to be taught to new members as the correct way to perceive, think, and feel in relation to those problems."[2, pp.373,374] These values can be observed in the behaviors the members of the group exhibit. New members learn the culture by picking up cues about what acceptable behavior is and what is not. Newcomers can react to the group culture by (1) acting the way the majority acts, (2) working to change the culture, (3) existing as an oddball, or (4) leaving.

WHAT IS A "CULTURE OF SAFETY"?

Nearly a decade after the Institute of Medicine report *To Err Is Human,*[3] in which a number of serious problems regarding the delivery of health care were identified, including the avoidable death of between 48,000 and 98,000 patients per year, there is a general consensus that change has been frustratingly slow.[4] The heart of the problem seems to be in the culture of health care, namely a lack of necessary characteristics within the culture that would likely lead to improvement. Other industries, those identified as "highly reliable," have developed a number of cultural characteristics that, when manifested, are believed to lead to a safer and therefore more reliable performance.[5,6] These highly reliable organizations foster a culture of safety because they develop "mindfulness" in their leaders, employees, staff, and team members.[5,6] This mindfulness has five essential components: a constant concern of the possibility of failure, deference to expertise regardless of rank or status, an ability to adapt when the unexpected occurs, an ability to concentrate on a specific task (including the development of a shared mental model among team members) while having a sense of the bigger picture and a broad awareness of the unfolding situation in the area (cross-monitoring and situational awareness), and an ability to alter and flatten organizational hierarchy as best fits the situation.[5,6] As the science of patient safety advances, health care's roads to such mindfulness and high reliability are coming into focus. Among the essential building blocks of a culture of safety in health care are (1) a fair and just culture for all involved, (2) leadership engagement, and (3) systematic and reinforced training in teamwork and effective communication.[7–9]

A culture of safety, therefore, is one in which safety is highly valued and resulting behaviors reflect this value. One characteristic of a safety culture is that peers, supervisors, and patients reward behaviors aimed at preventing errors, whereas unsafe behaviors are discouraged by peer pressure and formal evaluation procedures. A second characteristic is that when an error is made, the person who recognizes the error feels free to report it without causing negative repercussions toward those who "made the error" or to himself or herself. No one person is blamed for the error. This characteristic is important because it allows the causes of the error to be analyzed so that similar errors can be prevented in the future.

THE IDEAL SAFETY CULTURE

In the ideal healthcare safety culture, giving health care is an error-prone endeavor, and healthcare professionals are at high risk for making errors.[10] Every person involved is encouraged to identify possible safety problems and solutions, engage in safe care behaviors, and report errors and near misses without fear of being blamed and punished. If change in policies, procedures, or equipment is needed, the leaders act to make the necessary changes.

Everyone, regardless of position, is encouraged to do whatever it takes to make sure every part of care and the environment is as safe as possible. A member of the cleaning staff may recognize that some aspect of the environment is not safe for the child who is hospitalized. A patient may question a medication that he or she is offered because it looks different. A student may find that two medications prescribed for a patient are listed as having an interaction. The group response to these findings in a culture of safety is that each one is valued and encouraged. This type of culture is called "participative."[11] Every level in the hierarchy is encouraged to participate in identifying potential safety problems and solutions and is rewarded for doing so.

When an error or near miss situation does occur in this ideal environment, the person who made the error or the one who recognizes it reports it. Steps are taken to investigate the circumstances thoroughly and identify the factors that led to the error. Changes are made in procedures, products, and training that will prevent that same error from happening again.

Values and Beliefs That Compete with the Valuing of Safety

All healthcare providers should have an interest in not making errors for their patients, their institutions, and their own peace of mind; however, safety is not always the highest priority value of a culture. It is not that healthcare providers have a conscious plan to provide unsafe care. Instead, being able to give care quickly and economically and even without too much hard work may take precedence over safety. Accomplishing these alternate goals is easier if everyone in the setting works toward them; thus, some caregivers may put pressure on others to adopt the alternate goals. The evidence suggests that in many healthcare institutions the culture has evolved so that safety-focused behaviors are less socially acceptable than competing behaviors. These behaviors include seeking out, blaming, and punishing staff member(s) involved in errors, autonomy among providers, a lack of teamwork, a lack of transparency about errors, and poor communication. Industry-wide problems include a lack of appropriate training in the science of human error and a professional code that requires "perfect" performance among providers, a lack of understanding of basic systems design and management, and inattention to clinical outcomes.

Taking time to verify an unclear order takes time. Completing tasks as quickly as possible may be valued more highly than being safe. Checking on an unclear order may be inconvenient for the person who wrote the order. Questioning an order that is clear but seems unsafe may be perceived as lack of respect for that person's clinical competence. Preserving the good will of those higher up in the hierarchy may be given a higher value than giving safe care. Reluctance to "make waves" may be an individual personality characteristic, but it may also be a cultural characteristic. It is somewhat like an ancient culture avoiding certain behaviors because they might "incur the wrath of the gods."

Another cultural characteristic that affects safety is the attitude toward following rules. Some cultures have the belief that "rules are made to be broken." It is acceptable in these cultures to ignore rules, especially if the rationale for the rule is unknown or not considered to have value. Spath illustrated this phenomenon with the example of the number of people who violate highway speed limits.[12] Although they are breaking a law that is intended to provide a safe driving environment, many people feel that it is acceptable to break this law because they do not see the value behind it. The same cultural phenomenon can occur in healthcare settings; if healthcare providers do not believe that a procedure will prevent errors, they may ignore it. As more technologies and procedures aimed at preventing errors become available, it will be important to change this attitude also so that caregivers do not develop "workarounds" that defeat the purpose.[13]

Effect of Healthcare Organization/Disorganization on Safety Culture

The complex organizational structure of an academic healthcare institution can lead to a mix of cultures operating within one patient care setting. Rather than being one tightly controlled hierarchy, like a manufacturing plant, several power structures often exist. A traditional healthcare institution usually has a power structure with top-level managers, mid-level managers, and "front-line" workers who are staff nurses, pharmacists, physical therapists, dietitians, and so forth; however, physicians are often part of a separate power structure that is headed by a medical director.[14] In addition, private physicians (and possibly other practitioners) can admit patients to the hospital and give orders concerning their care because they have "hospital privileges," which gives the institution only limited control over their practice. In an academic healthcare center, students and student groups participate in caring for patients, but these students and often their instructors are not actual members of the formal hierarchy. They may be bound by the same policies and procedures, but enforcement is more dependent on faculty.

The private physicians, students, and faculty are somewhat like "guests" in most care settings (e.g., hospitals, skilled nursing facilities). The amount of time that they spend in the setting varies but is often very short. Thus, they are likely not to be influenced by the culture of the setting itself and do not become acculturated to the same extent. The emphasis placed on safety behaviors may be entirely different from the institution in which they are practicing.

Effect of Professional Autonomy on Culture of Safety

Another factor that affects traditional power structures within healthcare settings is that most of those involved are professionals. Most healthcare professions have professional organizations with codes of ethics that emphasize safety in patient care (see the Chapter 2 discussion); however, professionals often believe they have professional autonomy to make decisions that they believe are in the best interest of their patients. They believe that only those who have the same professional credentials, often from a professional organization, have the right and responsibility to regulate them. Thus, policies regarding safety may or may not be followed because the professional may not believe himself or herself to be governed by them. A systematic educational approach to correcting this issue regarding providing safe care and coordinating the team has been proposed for physicians, and there is wide-spread belief that changing the culture of health care will take time and require a combination of education, peer review, licensure requirements, and organizational credentialing processes.[15]

REACTION TO ERRORS

An important aspect of a culture of safety is the group's reaction to a safety-related error or accident. Because healthcare providers value safe care, they may react to an error by blaming and punishing the person who committed it. It has been found that when an individual is blamed for an error, the tendency is for errors not to be reported and possibly even be hidden.[3] When errors or near misses are not reported, no investigation into what factors contributed to the error and no change in the environment or process occur. The same conditions continue to exist, and errors continue to happen.

The general American culture in which a healthcare organization exists also influences the culture of safety within the institution. A frequent reaction to an error is to want to find out who is responsible for making it and to make sure that the person is punished or pays for the damages. Americans are often considered litigious because of the tendency to want to sue another person when they feel they have been wronged. DeVille and Elliot noted that American beliefs have evolved from blaming witchcraft and supernatural powers for unfortunate events (even medical errors) to the current notion that a human being must be responsible for every error.[16]

BLAME-FREE CULTURE VERSUS JUST CULTURE

In a culture of safety, everyone must be willing to report errors, near misses, and unsafe situations. This is a "reporting culture."[17] The characteristics of the environment that might lead to this willingness to report, however, have been under discussion. As the Institute for Safe Medication Practices noted, the prevailing attitude regarding errors could be characterized as a "punitive culture" until the 1990s.[18] In this punitive culture, those who made errors were disciplined or at least "counseled" with the goal of preventing errors from happening; however, the punitive culture interfered with the reporting culture. Thus, instead of preventing errors, it led to more errors.

The reaction to this realization in the 1990s led to the proposal of a blame-free culture, in which no individual is ever blamed for an error.[18] The rationale for this is that when people fear being blamed and possibly punished for something, they are not as likely to report errors. Not all have accepted the idea of errors being totally blame free because there are situations in which individuals should be accountable.[17]

The Institute for Safe Medication Practices has asserted that the pendulum has swung from a punitive culture to a blame-free culture and has now come to the midpoint: a "just culture."[19] A just culture is one that is fair to those who make an error but does not give amnesty to all. Errors are analyzed for individual accountability as well as for the contribution of the system to the error.[17] Culpability of an individual may be found to be present if the person committed an unsafe act deliberately, was knowingly reckless, or was impaired through substance abuse.[19]

MEASURING THE CULTURE OF SAFETY IN HOSPITALS

In 2004, the Agency for Healthcare Research and Quality (AHRQ) published the Patient Safety Culture Survey, which measures healthcare providers' opinions about the culture of safety in their practice areas. The questions in this survey reflect several dimensions of the culture of safety: (1) attitudes that are held within a work unit, (2) behaviors of the unit manager, (3) communications that affect safety, (4) frequency of reporting of mistakes, (5) opinion about the entire hospital's safety culture, and (6) an opportunity to give the work unit a patient safety grade.[20]

The AHRQ encourages hospitals to use a tool like this to "measure" the culture of safety on an annual basis so that progress toward improving that culture can be assessed. Data from this type of survey also assist in decisions about which aspect of the culture needs to be improved and perhaps which unit has the highest priority need for improvement. In addition, use of the AHRQ survey allows hospitals to "benchmark" their results (compare the responses of their staffs with responses at other hospitals) because the AHRQ provides survey results from hospitals who voluntarily share their data.

2007 Culture of Safety Survey Results

The survey results shared on the AHRQ site give an overall picture of the present status of the culture of safety in American hospitals.[21] As these results are reviewed, keep in mind that they may be biased because they were voluntarily submitted and hospitals who found that their culture of safety was poor may have been reluctant to share their results. Thus, these results may show a better picture than actually exists. Although the hospitals that participated were not selected by sampling so that they could be considered representative of all U.S. hospitals, the AHRQ stated that the characteristics of the hospitals are consistent with the distribution of hospitals in the United States.

The 2007 Comparative Database includes data from 108,621 staff members in 382 hospitals.[21] These hospitals were large and small, private and government owned, and were located in every region of the country; thus, these data give us some kind of an idea what the status of the culture of safety really is in American hospitals. The summarized results are available on the AHRQ website.[21]

The results show that respondents were most positive about "teamwork within units"—the extent to which staff support each other, treat each other with respect, and works as a team. In this category, 78% of the respondents gave a positive response.[21]

This attitude is important for a culture of safety because hospital staff members often need help, and not having it available could lead to unsafe conditions. In addition to helping each other, however, "supporting each other" could also mean that they do not report each other's mistakes. The responses were not so high for "teamwork across units," an area that only 57% rated in a positive way.[21]

Another interesting comparison is between ratings attributed to administrators and management and those that are not in these positions. The ratings from administrators were higher for all of the categories, than most other staff members. For example, in the category of "management support of patient safety," 82% of the administrative raters gave positive ratings, whereas only 64% of the nursing staff was on the positive side. A response to one particular item about management was as follows: "Hospital management seems interested in patient safety only after an adverse event happens." This shows the difference in perceptions. Ratings from administrators on this negatively worded item were 74% positive. This means that 74% disagreed with it; however, ratings from all other categories of workers ranged from 54% to 61%.[21]

The lowest ratings were in the category labeled "nonpunitive response to error," which measured perceptions being blame free. The items included the extent to which staff members felt that mistakes are held against them and recorded in their personnel files, and reports about the event indicated that the person rather than the event was the problem. In this category, only 43% were positive.[21]

In this safety culture survey, the respondents were asked to give a safety grade from A (Excellent) to E (Failing) to their work area or unit. The 2007 results from the 108,000 respondents reveal that about 70% of these staff members gave their work areas an A or B. Only 6% felt that the safety grade was less than acceptable.[21]

Comparison Between 2007 Results and 2008 Results

The 2008 results of the Patient Safety Culture Survey include data from 98 hospitals that conducted the safety culture survey in both 2007 and 2008.[22] This type of trending is valuable in seeing whether there is an improvement in the culture of safety over time. These preliminary results show that in these 98 hospitals some had increases in their positive ratings, some had decreases in positive ratings, and many stayed the same. Overall, it appears that the increases outnumber the decreases. For example, for the "nonpunitive response to error" category, 38% of the hospitals had an increase of at least 5% in positive response, 16% had a decrease of at least 5%, and 45% stayed the same (did not change more than 5%).[22]

Although the results of these surveys are interesting and give us an overall view, the greater value is for administrators of individual hospitals to know how their facility compares with others and how it changes over time. The results also help them to see staff perceptions of the culture of safety, rather than only using their own perceptions. Thus, as they attempt to improve the culture of safety, they can see whether the outcomes show that their efforts made a difference.

CHANGING TO A SAFETY CULTURE— TOP DOWN AND BOTTOM UP

Culture develops over time and cannot be mandated by management; however, managers can have a profound effect on the culture of safety. Managers can affect behavior by providing informal positive feedback for safety-focused behaviors and by providing negative feedback for behaviors that are not safe. Formal evaluation and the granting or withholding of promotions and salary increases are powerful motivators. If managers reward staff members who spend time ensuring safety over those who complete their work on time, safety behaviors will thrive.[23]

Leaders of an institution who want to encourage a culture of safety must make their interest in safety clear and widely known. They need to make safety part of their mission and goals and to find ways to communicate that they are serious. Whittington and Cohen described "executive walkarounds" in which the executive visits patient care areas and asks workers questions about safety problem concerns that they have noticed.[24] This practice helps to identify safety problems and shows the workers that management is interested in safety and their knowledge of safety. Managers must also make certain that a specific policy is in place in case an error is made. This policy must state that the person who makes the error is not blamed and punished. It must also outline steps to identify the cause of the error and correct it.

Management can influence the safety culture by providing the resources needed to improve it. Safety should be considered in all equipment and procedure decisions. Time for developing better safety procedures and time for training workers in safety procedures need to be financed. When leaders not only say they value safety but provide the resources to develop a culture of safety, the employees are much more likely to value safety.

Culture change also needs to occur "from the bottom up," however. Healthcare workers need to take personal responsibility for ensuring that safe care is the norm in their setting and take steps to change procedures if they are not safe. Each individual needs to espouse the blame-free attitude to errors and report their own errors and other unsafe behavior and errors that they see others make. Although being a "tattletale" or "snitch" is generally considered as showing disloyalty to the group,[25] individuals need to be able to be confident that bringing an error to attention will help prevent that error from occurring in the future.

STRATEGIES AND TOOLS FOR CHANGING TO A CULTURE OF SAFETY

Changing to a culture of safety is not a simple, easy process. Rose, Thomas, Tersigni, Sexton, and Pryor have described their efforts to do this in an article describing the "Five C's of Culture Change."[26] The first C is "comprehension," understanding the problem. The safety culture surveys help with this, but these authors pointed out that "mutual comprehension" is needed—not just comprehension by the administrators and not just understanding that there is a problem, but also understanding what is causing the problem and how each person and profession fits in.

The second C is "compassion."[26] This is associated with the creation of a non-punitive culture, in which mistakes are system problems. These authors also included being emotionally open to change, a characteristic that is necessary for caregivers to admit that the way they have been practicing might not be the best way for patient safety.

The third C is "collaboration."[26] Collaboration needs to be between subcultures and care providers of different professions and levels of authority. The authors suggested that staff members need to be able to feel enough "psychological safety" to suggest innovative ideas, to critique others and accept critiques by others, and to take ownership of errors.

The fourth C is "coordination."[26] Coordination involves communication and information flow. The emphasis is on standardization in data, terminology, and processes to minimize errors caused by a lack of communication.

The fifth C is "convergence."[26] This last element emphasizes the need to work together to become safety oriented in all situations. The goal would be to make safety orientation the new norm for healthcare institutions.

TEAMSTEPPS: TOOLS FOR A CULTURE OF SAFETY

A more specific set of tools for developing a culture of safety and safe communication procedures is called TeamSTEPPS, developed by the Department of Defense in collaboration with the AHRQ.[27] TeamSTEPPS is an evidence-based curriculum made publicly available in November of 2006 and has been used widely within the military and other government healthcare organizations.[28] According to the Military Health System,[29] TeamSTEPPS transforms culture in five ways: (1) It establishes names for behaviors and a common language for talking about failure of communication, (2) it bridges the professional divide and levels the hierarchy, (3) it provides "actions" to practice, (4) it increases mindfulness, and (5) it enlists the patient as a valued team member.

One of the major principles of TeamSTEPPS is mutual support among team members in which the members are asked to protect each other from work overload situations that do not support patient safety.[27] The idea is to foster a culture in which asking for assistance is expected and in which assistance will be offered when needed to give safe care. Mutual support also includes the expectation that each team member will act as an advocate for the patient when he or she believes that another member of the team has made a decision that affects patient safety. According to AHRQ, this principle "empowers all team members to 'stop the line' if they sense or discover an essential safety breach."[30, p.23] TeamSTEPPS provides mnemonic tools for team members to use to bring up these concerns. The specific one for a suspected safety breach is "CUS," which stands for "I am *C*oncerned! I am *U*ncomfortable! This is a *S*afety issue!"[30, p.24]

Another TeamSTEPPS principle that is closely related to the culture of safety is situation monitoring.[30] This principle encourages team members to monitor the actions of other team members to assure that patient safety is maintained. This is a significant change in culture from the one in which some professionals believed that they were responsible for only their own actions. In addition, each team member is responsible for monitoring whether his or her own attention to patient safety might be impaired. The mnemonic used for monitoring this is "IMSAFE," which encourages the team member to pay attention to impairment caused by illness, medication, stress, alcohol and drugs, fatigue, and eating and elimination.

Other principles advanced in the TeamSTEPPS curriculum are communication, leadership, team structure, and the critical importance of the change process that is required whenever a new training program is brought into an organization.[31]

SUMMARY

A culture of safety is one in which patient safety is valued above all else. Among the many barriers to establishing a culture of safety is the possibility of individual punishment when reporting an error. Recent surveys of the culture of safety in

American hospitals illustrate room for improvement. Strategies are being developed to encourage a development of a culture to improve patient safety.

A CLOSING CASE

Read the following case, and use the questions that follow to apply what you have learned in this chapter:

Joan W. is a registered nurse who has worked on a surgical unit for 10 years. Dr. B. is a surgeon whose patients come to this unit for postoperative care. Joan has never known Dr. B. to make an error or had any reason to question any of his orders. One day Dr. B. came to the unit at 7:30 p.m. after an especially long and hard day in the operating room. He looked very tired and said he thought he was getting the flu. He wrote a long set of orders for a postoperative hip fracture patient, but he did not include an order for Lovenox, as he usually did. Joan did not notice the omission until 11:30 p.m. She wondered whether he could have forgotten the order because he was so tired and possibly sick, but she did not want to call him because it was so late. She told herself that there are contraindications to Lovenox and that Dr. B probably had a good reason for not ordering it. Joan saw Dr. B in the morning as he made his 6 a.m. rounds before surgery, but by that time, she was so tired she forgot to ask about the Lovenox.

Tom F. is a junior nursing student assigned to care for the patient starting at 7 a.m. the next morning. When he had been at the hospital the evening before to gather information for his plan of care, the patient's orders were not available yet. When he saw the orders in the morning, he wondered why there was no order for deep vein thrombosis (DVT) prevention because it was included in the clinical practice guideline. When he took the report from Joan W., he asked her. This reminded her that she meant to ask Dr. B., and, before she left, she called down to the operating room and had a nurse ask Dr. B about it. He responded that he must have forgotten it, gave a verbal order, and the patient received the first dose of Lovenox on the first postoperative day as the protocol specified. The patient recovered well and had no evidence of a DVT. Dr. B. told Joan later that he was so glad that she had reminded him about the need for a Lovenox order.

1. If Tom had not asked about the omission and the patient developed a DVT, whose fault would it have been?
2. If Dr. B. had previously rebuffed Joan for asking him questions about omissions in orders, might that have prevented her from calling him?

3. If Joan had told Tom that she was not going to ask because she knew Dr. B. well and that he never made mistakes, what should he have done?
4. What system features could have been used to make sure that an order like this was not forgotten?
5. Would it be appropriate to report this event as a near miss? Is this just an everyday occurrence?
6. What other professionals might have been in a position to catch this error of omission?

Discussion Questions to Launch Further Investigation

For further investigation, seek answers to these questions:

1. Describe a situation you have seen (or can imagine) in which something else was valued higher than giving the safest care possible.
2. If you were a health professional working in an environment where you see a culture that is not a culture of safety, what would you do?
3. Does "blame free" mean that health professionals should never be held accountable and disciplined for errors?
4. Describe a situation in which you think a healthcare professional might be reluctant to point out a potential error to another professional.

REFERENCES

1. Newman DM. *Sociology: Exploring the Architecture of Everyday Life*, 3rd ed. Thousand Oaks, CA: Pine Forge Press; 2000.
2. Schein E. Organizational culture and leadership. In: Shafritz JM, Ott JS, eds. *Classics of Organization Theory*. Fort Worth, TX: Harcourt; 1993.
3. Kohn LT, Corrigan JM, Donaldson MS, eds. *To Err Is Human: Building a Safer Health System*. Washington, DC: National Academy Press; 2000.
4. Leape LL, Berwick DM. Five years after *To Err Is Human*: what have we learned? *JAMA* 2005;293:2384–2390.
5. Roberts KH. Cultural characteristics of reliability enhancing organizations. *J Manage Issues* 1993;5:165–181.
6. Weick K, Sutcliffe K. *Managing the Unexpected: Assuring High Performance in an Age of Complexity*. San Francisco, CA: Jossey-Bass; 2001.
7. Gaba DM. Structural and organizational issues in patient safety: a comparison of health care to other high-hazard industries. *Calif Manage Rev* 2000;43:83–102.
8. Helmreich RL. On error management: lessons from aviation. *Br Med J* 2000;320:781–785.
9. Leonard M, Graham S, Bonacum D. The human factor: the critical importance of effective teamwork and communication in providing safe care. *Qual Saf Health Care* 2004;13(Suppl 1):i85–i90.
10. Pizzi LT, Goldfarb NI, Nash DB. Promoting a culture of safety. In *Making Health Care Safer: A Critical Analysis of Patient Safety Practices*. Evidence Report/Technology Assessment:

Number 43. AHRQ Publication No. 01-E058, July 2001. Agency for Healthcare Research and Quality, Rockville, MD. Available at: http://www.ahrq.gov/clinic/ptsafety/. Accessed March 28, 2009.

11. Wakefield BJ, Blegen MA, Uden-Holman TU, Vaughn T, Chrischilles E, Wakefield DS. Organizational culture, continuous quality improvement, and medication administration error reporting. *Am J Med Qual* 2001;16:128–134.

12. Spath PL. It's Time for a Patient Safety Culture Revolution, 2002. Available at: http://www.brownspath.com/original_articles/culture.htm. Accessed March 28, 2009.

13. AHRQ PSNet Patient Safety Network. Agency for Healthcare Research and Quality Web site. Available at http://www.psnet.ahrq.gov/glossary.aspx#W. Accessed March 28, 2009.

14. Pernal-Wallag MS. Safety culture. In: *University of Michigan Health System Patient Safety Toolkit*. Available at: http://www.med.umich.edu/patientsafetytoolkit/culture/chapter.pdf. Accessed March 28, 2009.

15. Baker DP, Salas E, King H, Battles J, Barach P. The role of teamwork in the professional education of physicians: current status and assessment recommendations. *Jt Comm J Qual Patient Saf* 2005;31:185–202.

16. DeVille K, Elliott C. To err is human: American culture, history, and medical error. In Rubin SB, Zoloth L, eds. *Margin of Error: The Ethics of Mistakes in the Practice of Medicine*. Hagerstown, MD: University Publishing Group; 2000.

17. AORN. AORN guidance statement: Creating a patient safety culture. *AORN J* 2006; 83:936–942.

18. Institute for Safe Medication Practices. Our long journey towards a safety-minded just culture. Part I: Where we've been. *ISMP Newsletter*. September 7, 2006. Available at: http://www.ismp.org/newsletters/acutecare/articles/20060907.asp. Accessed March 29, 2009.

19. Institute for Safe Medication Practices. Our long journey towards a safety-minded just culture. Part II: Where we're going. ISMP Newsletter. September 21, 2006. Available at: http://www.ismp.org/newsletters/acutecare/articles/20060921.asp. Accessed March 29, 2009.

20. Patient Safety Culture Surveys, March 2009. Agency for Healthcare Research and Quality, Rockville, MD. Available at: http://www.ahrq.gov/qual/patientsafetyculture/. Accessed March 29, 2009.

21. *Hospital Survey on Patient Safety Culture: 2007 Comparative Database Report*. AHRQ Publication No. 07-0025, April 2007. Agency for Healthcare Research and Quality, Rockville, MD. Available at: http://www.ahrq.gov/qual/hospsurveydb/. Accessed March 29, 2009.

22. *Hospital Survey on Patient Safety Culture: 2008 Comparative Database Report*. AHRQ Publication No. 08-0039, March 2008. Agency for Healthcare Research and Quality, Rockville, MD. Available at: http://www.ahrq.gov/qual/hospsurvey08. Accessed March 29, 2009.

23. Ruchlin HS. The role of leadership in instilling a culture of safety: lessons from the literature. *J Healthcare Manage* 2004;49:47–58.

24. Whittington J, Cohen H. OSF Healthcare's journey in patient safety. *Qual Manage Health Care* 2004;13:53–59.

25. Darr K. Tattletales, culture, and quality of care. *Hosp Top* 1997;75:4–8.

26. Rose JS, Thomas CS, Tersigni A, Sexton JB, Pryor D. A leadership framework for culture change in health care. *Jt Comm J Qual Patient Saf* 2006;32:433–442.

27. Agency for Healthcare Research and Quality. TeamSTEPPS: National Implementation. Available at: http://teamstepps.ahrq.gov/index.htm. Accessed March 29, 2009.

28. Clancy CM, Tornberg DN. TeamSTEPPS: Integrating teamwork principles into healthcare practice. Patient Safety and Quality Healthcare e-Newsletter. November/December, 2006. Available at: http://www.psqh.com/novdec06/ahrq.html. Accessed March 29, 2009.

29. Military Health System. TeamSTEPPS. Paper presented at: 2008 MHS Conference; January 28–31, 2008; Washington, DC. Available at: http://www.health.mil/conferences/2008MHS/downloads/W_1530%20TeamSTEPPS%20Training%20083.ppt. Accessed March 29, 2009.

30. Agency for Healthcare Research and Quality. *TeamSTEPPS Pocket Guide: Strategies & Tools to Enhance Performance and Patient Safety.* Rockville, MD: Department of Defense and Agency for Healthcare Research and Quality; 2006.

31. Kotter J, Rathgeber H. *Our Iceberg Is Melting: Changing and Succeeding Under Any Conditions.* New York: St. Martin's Press; 2006.

CHAPTER 7

Why Things Go Wrong

Kimberly A. Galt, Kevin T. Fuji, John M. Gleason,
and Robert J. McQuillan

PURPOSE

The purpose of this chapter is to provide fundamental knowledge about the science of errors. An understanding of the inherent nature of errors is needed to improve human performance and structure considerations in safety.

OBJECTIVES

After completing this chapter, the student will be able to:

- Analyze how errors occur as a result of cognitive, psychosocial, environmental, and task-related factors
- Describe the scope, causes, and types of errors and the outcomes that result
- Describe how our understanding of human performance fallibility is approached in the design of safe systems
- Explain the relevance of human factors and the science of human error, performance, and systems engineering to efforts to improve patient safety
- Explain how clinical environments such as the operating room can use the science of human factors and a systems approach to understand errors to improve safety in health care

VIGNETTE

A few years ago, my brother John was complaining about headaches, fever, and body aches (especially in his lower back). He started taking Advil, but within a week, he also began experiencing painful urination, leading him to schedule a physician visit.

We had recently switched healthcare providers, and this was John's first visit with our new physician. My brother thought the doctor seemed nice; however, he seemed stressed, rushed, and distracted. After the doctor listened to my brother's symptoms, he performed a quick checkup. He immediately diagnosed John as having a simple infection and declared that the Advil was causing his painful urination. My brother told him he had taken Advil for years and had never experienced a problem with it before. The doctor brushed off my brother's concerns, prescribed some antibiotics and a pain reliever, and dismissed him. The entire interaction took about 5 minutes.

Over the following week John's symptoms worsened, and he called the physician. The doctor assured him that he would get better as long as he kept taking his medication. During the subsequent week, however, my brother's pain became excruciating and debilitating. After spending 2 days in bed, he drove himself to the emergency room, even though he could barely walk. Some testing was done, and it was discovered that John was suffering from kidney stones.

My brother became extremely angry with his primary care physician. After doing his own research, my brother noted that all of his symptoms could be explained by kidney stones. He discovered that some families were predisposed to developing kidney stones; had the doctor asked for a family history regarding this, he would have found that both of my parents and nearly all of the adults on my mother's side had suffered from kidney stones at some point in their lives. John accused the doctor of being negligent and believed that he jumped to conclusions because of his lack of attention and care. My brother never saw that doctor again and has developed a certain level of cynicism toward physicians.

ERRORS, MISTAKES, AND ACCIDENTS

Scope

For over 40 years, recurring evidence has shown that a large number of patients suffer injuries as a result of treatment while hospitalized.[1–3] The Harvard Medical Practice Study provided one of the most methodologically correct and comprehensive views of the scope of the problem.[4–7] The study focused on iatrogenic injuries to patients hospitalized in the state of New York in 1984. Approximately 4% of patients suffered serious iatrogenic injuries that lengthened their time in the hospital or resulted in disability; moreover, nearly 14% of these injuries were fatal.[6,7] Leape noted that if these rates were representative of those in the entire United States, iatrogenic injury would contribute to approximately 180,000 deaths each year—the equivalent of three jumbo-jet crashes every 2 days! The public would certainly demand immediate corrective action if faced with this level of aviation-related deaths. Because most healthcare-related deaths occur one at a time and in thousands of different locations, however, the issue does not cause a similar level of public outrage.

Most (69%) of the iatrogenic injuries were the result of errors. Errors can be defined as "the failure of a planned action to be completed as intended or the use of a wrong plan to achieve an aim."[8] The large number of iatrogenic injuries has even more troublesome implications relative to medical errors. Because most errors do not result in injuries, the large number of injuries documented in the Harvard study suggests a significantly larger number of medical errors.

The error rate in the practice of medicine is high for two primary reasons: a lack of awareness of the problem and the fact that most errors do no harm. A lack of awareness stems from the fact that medical errors are generally not reported in the media, like plane crashes. Although error rates are high, serious injuries are not part of the daily experience of physicians, nurses, and other healthcare professionals; instead, they are perceived as isolated and unusual events. People are rarely harmed because the errors either are intercepted or the patient's own defenses prevent injury. Many experts believe that the most important reason lies within the culture of medical practice itself: the difficulty of dealing with the reality of human error.[8]

Causes

Two basic types of medical errors exist: human and system errors. Human errors result from cognitive limitations. The causes for human errors may include accidents resulting from diversion of attention or the use of inappropriate heuristics in the decision-making process. In many instances, however, the root cause of human error is poor system design. Health care is a system, one that is complex and consists of many interconnected processes designed to achieve a common goal: getting the patient better. System design failures, however, make it very difficult, if not impossible, to reverse an error before it causes harm. Remember that every system is perfectly designed to achieve exactly the result it gets.

Historically, the medical approach to error prevention has been reactive and has focused on the individual. Training, education, protocols, and knowledge have been the focus of attempts to reduce human errors. If an error does occur, efforts are made to identify the *proximate cause* of the error (typically something an individual has or has not done) and to correct that cause. The correction effort may include increased emphasis on training and education with respect to the cause of the error; however, the *root cause*, that is, the system-related cause of the error, is seldom identified.[7]

The field of human factors provides substantial guidance about how to improve our understanding of the interactions between and among humans and other elements of a system and how to use our knowledge to improve the design, implementation, and use of various systems. When we describe the involvement of humans in this interaction in health care, we are inclusive of healthcare professionals and health-related workers who may be directly or indirectly involved in the delivery of care to patients, their families, and their caregivers. The human characteristics that can be considered relevant in understanding and applying human factors approaches include cognitive, physical, and psychosocial characteristics.[9] You will read more about these as we progress through this chapter.

Fortunately, in recent years, the fact that most errors result from system failures is becoming more recognized; therefore, a commitment to patient safety requires a simultaneous commitment to system design, maintenance, and operation, similar to that of the engineering disciplines. Appropriate systems can be expected to reduce the probability of human errors within those systems.

Systems can be thought of as having two different levels. One level is the work system, which designs systems to prevent errors (or make them less likely), designs procedures to make errors more visible when they do occur, and designs procedures to mitigate the effects of errors when they occur and are not caught before reaching the patient. The second level is the management system, which focuses on designing and creating the work system and its subsequent maintenance, redesign, and change.

Types of Errors

It is important to distinguish between potential errors and actual errors. Potential errors are mostly systems-related errors that result from poor systems design, maintenance, and operation. Leape and Reason called this type of error a *latent error*, the root cause of which has existed in the system for some time.[7,10] They noted that the individual who is the proximate cause of the actual error that ultimately occurs has been set up to fail by the system. The Three Mile Island nuclear meltdown incident is a good example of how latent errors in a system will eventually lead to an actual error. Latent errors result from decisions at the higher echelons of organizations; they may lie dormant for long periods of time, eventually becoming evident when they combine with triggering factors that lead to adverse consequences. In the Three Mile Island incident, latent errors included poor human equipment interfaces (workers did not understand the actual meaning of an indicator light due to ambiguity), poor maintenance of equipment, and poor training/education. Other examples of latent errors are understaffing, high workload, or poor management/leadership.

Actual errors may result from latent errors or from limitations of human cognition; that is, actual errors may be system errors or human errors. In some instances, a latent error leads to an actual error because of tight coupling within the system (see Chapter 1). The interactive complexity of the system may lead to an unexpected occurrence, and there is not the time and/or a means to intervene before the unexpected event causes an actual error. Figure 7–1 shows how system errors occur when we consider these in the context of the organization, workplace, and individual persons involved. This model is used to illustrate that when individuals are involved in accidental events that lead to harm and injury, they are generally set up to fail by the surrounding organization and workplace system factors.

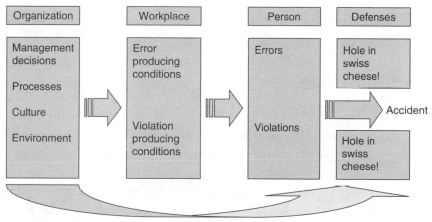

Latent failure pathway

FIGURE 7–1 The Latent Failure Pathway That Describes an Accident in an Organization

Adapted from Reason J, Hobbs A. *Managing Maintenance Error: A Practical Guide.* Burlington, VT: Ashgate Publishing Company; 2003.

Outcomes

An indication of the harm caused by medical errors was noted previously—iatrogenic injuries contribute to approximately 180,000 deaths each year.[7] Moreover, a more recent MedPAC Report to Congress indicates that hundreds of thousands of Medicare beneficiaries experience adverse events each year.[11]

Further evidence of the magnitude of the problem of medical errors is provided by Zhan and Miller.[12] They used the Agency for Healthcare Research and Quality Patient Safety Indicators in an examination of more than 7 million hospital discharge abstracts from a sample of approximately 20% of U.S. hospitals. By extrapolating their findings, they determined that medical errors result in more than 32,000 deaths and $9.3 billion in excess medical charges annually in the United States.

HUMAN ERROR

Errors occur in our world because neither humans nor machines are perfect. In health care, as in all organizations or industries, humans and machines perform tasks and carry out functions, processes, and activities that collectively lead to a certain level of performance. Human and technological performance over time create measurable outcomes. When measured and compared with an expected or required level of performance, the undeniable effect of error on performance becomes apparent. In the world of organizational performance, some industries have been working on these issues for decades in an effort to deliver intended and expected outcomes more reliably (e.g., the nuclear power industry, NASA, aviation, high-speed rail, and the military). When an organization can demonstrate a level of safe and effective performance that is considered to be as close as possible to the ideal, it is referred to as a "high-reliability organization." A number of characteristics of high-reliability organizations contribute to a near-perfect level of performance, but at the core of the culture of such organizations lies an in-depth understanding and appreciation of the human factors involved in the generation of errors and how to manage the issues involved to maximize human performance. These organizations have learned that knowledge of human strengths and limitations can lead to better system design, more effective training, and better assessment of the usability of the system.

In order to understand better a near-perfect level of performance, consider an intensive care unit study that revealed that patients received an average of 178 "activities" each day (all with the potential for iatrogenic harm) with an average of 1.7 errors per day.[13] This number of errors likely does not seem large, and indeed, it equates to a 99% level of proficiency; however, even a 1% error rate is substantially higher than other high-risk industries such as aviation and nuclear power would tolerate.

Deming once noted that if we had to live with 99.9% proficiency in other industries we would have two unsafe landings each day at O'Hare International Airport, 16,000 pieces of lost mail every hour, and 32,000 bank checks that would be deducted from the wrong bank account every hour![7] All of a sudden a 99% level of proficiency in health care does not seem so safe!

Human Factors Approach to Errors

Humans are very good at learning and performing tasks, especially those we are faced with frequently. We excel at learning in an adaptive fashion, and thus, the more routine and common a certain task is, the better our brain and neuromuscular system adapt to reduce the amount of energy required (both cognitive and physical). In some sense, as we adapt, the more technically "expert" we become at a given task, the less taxing it will be. This remarkable ability to adapt to the environment and become extremely efficient at the skills and tasks needed for survival is the core of all existence. These same basic mechanisms are involved whether referring to the most common human tasks such as walking down the street or the not so common tasks such as brain surgery. The relationship between automatic actions and those that we must consciously perform has been shown in relationship to how routine that action is. The less routine, or more novel, the action, the more problematic this is for human beings. When humans perform these different actions, the person's performance can be identified and described as skill, rule, or knowledge based. This is displayed in a matrix shown in Table 7–1 adapted from the work of Reason, Hobbs, and Rasmussen.[14,15] The discussion that follows provides a greater understanding of this human action framework to inform us about the nature of how it is that humans are "wired" to make errors.

As humans become more expert at a given task, the cognitive adaptive mechanisms allow for an "auto-pilot" mode of cognitive performance. A simple example of this is driving a car. Compare the first time a person drives a car in his or her mid-teens to the capability of that same person after 10 years of driving. The former is exhausting, requiring a great deal of attention and effort, whereas the latter is "auto-pilot," with a part of the brain more in "monitoring" mode while our minds and neuromuscular systems carry out most of the work without much thought. Driving at this level becomes routine, almost effortless, and even allows us to conduct other activities at the same time, such as carrying on conversations, singing to the radio, talking on a cell phone, or thinking about an upcoming job

Table 7–1 Relationship of Human Performance Level to Situations and Behavioral Control Modes

Situations		Control Modes		
		Conscious • Slow • Effortful • Limited • Sequential • Universal • New tasks	Mixed	Automatic • Rapid • Effortless • Unlimited • Parallel • Specific • Skilled tasks
Less Problematic	Routine • Familiar • Predictable • Frequent • Feels comfortable			Skill-based performance Automatic control of routine tasks with occasional checks on progress.
	Expected and trained for problems		Rule-based performance Pattern-matching prepared rules or solutions to trained-for problems.	
More Problematic	Novel problems • Unfamiliar • Unexpected • Rare • Can be frightening	Knowledge-based performance Conscious, slow, effortful attempts to solve new problems online.		

Adapted from Reason J, Hobbs A. *Managing Maintenance Error: A Practical Guide.* Burlington, VT: Ashgate Publishing Company; 2003.

activity. Countless examples exist of this profound human capability in everyday life. Even brain surgery becomes "routine" for the experienced neurosurgeon.

This human performance and the remarkable capacity for taking complex tasks and making them routine and "automatic" has a downside. It is critical to understand this clearly when considering human error, human performance, and complex environments such as health care. James Reason puts it very well in his book *Human Error*[10, p.17]:

> The more predictable varieties of human fallibility are rooted in the essential and adaptive properties of human cognition. They are the penalties that must be paid for our remarkable ability to model the regularities of the world and then to use these stored representations to simplify complex information-handling tasks. They represent the debit side of the cognitive "balance sheet," where each entry also carries significant advantages.

Human factors engineering is the study of factors and the development of tools that facilitate the improvement of human interaction with systems. The goal is to make the human interaction with systems one that reduces error, increases productivity, and enhances safety and reliability.

Humans are adaptively engineered to prefer to be in the automatic mode of performance most of the time. This has huge implications for error-reduction efforts because it means that many experts carry out much of their task-related activities in "auto-pilot" and therefore don't pay attention to the little details related to the task, leading to a very predictable set of errors that are routine and expected. Such errors occur in everyday life and in high-risk industries as well. The important message here is this: Most errors that occur in human experience cannot be prevented. Thus, what can we do so this never happens again? Systems must be designed to recognize when the errors are likely to occur and to provide support in the form of alerting those involved, correcting the action, or providing some form of mitigation so as to prevent the error from causing harm. To create effective error-reduction strategies, an understanding of these "human factors" is essential.

Humans should not be expected to just rely on memory, rely on vigilance, or expect excellent performance when fatigued or stressed. Techniques, tools, strategies to reduce errors, and monitoring methods for a successful reduction and avoidance of errors are important to incorporate into our daily work in health care. Additionally, we must also deal with design flaws in health care, including naming, packaging, and labeling; handwriting; matching staffing with demand; medication delivery; accepting mediocre performance; "sort and shoot" approaches to error (e.g., focusing on identifying and then blaming individuals instead of using a systems approach); and complexity. Techniques widely used in a variety of industries to address potential patient safety problems include simplifying and standardizing (e.g., checklists and other forms of memory aids, processes to assist in precision during "mission critical processes"), reducing handoffs and formally structuring communication processes, eliminating redundancy, "forcing" functions, and using team training and technology.

The study of cognitive psychology has identified three cognitive models of performance: schematic control, rule based, and attention control. The schematic control model is also known as skill based and is unconscious, rapid, and effortless (e.g., driving home on a familiar route). The rule-based model is predicated on a series of actions: if x, then y (e.g., if it rains, then you pull out an umbrella). The attention control model is knowledge based and requires novel problem solving (e.g., completing a problem that you have not previously encountered).

When humans make errors, the errors can be classified as either a slip or a mistake. Slips are skill based, whereas mistakes are rule or knowledge based. Slips are the most common error because much of our mental functioning is automatic. Slips occur more frequently with fatigue, illness, alcohol, sleep deprivation, boredom, fear, anxiety, stress, and environmental distractions (e.g., noise, heat, motion).

Although slips are the most common type of error, mistakes occur more frequently than slips. Two types of mistakes exist: rule-based errors and knowledge-based errors. Rule-based errors stem from application of the wrong rule, misapplication of the correct rule, or nonapplication of the correct rule. Knowledge-based errors consist of biased memory, availability heuristic (tendency to use the first information that comes to mind), confirmation bias (a tendency to look for evidence supporting an early hypothesis, even if it is wrong), and overconfidence.

Some of the ways we understand human limitations are described here:

Inherent human limitations. Physical, cognitive, and psychosocial characteristics of people establish our boundaries for safety. The work environment can impose physical stresses on workers. Systems to deliver care should be designed around a thorough understanding of physical human characteristics, such as height, weight, reading level, physical strength, and physical movement, and senses, such as vision, hearing, smell, taste, and touch. Better systems will use guiding principles for such things as workspace layout, equipment, and technologies. These principles include minimizing detection and perception time, minimizing decision time, minimizing manipulation time, and optimizing opportunity for movement.

Stress. Stress in healthcare employment has been identified most closely to burnout and accidents among healthcare workers. The physical stress of lifting repeatedly at work is a predictor of burnout and significant for job stress and self-rated poorer health. Being threatened on the job is the single best predictor of accidents and present among many workers who report burnout. Insufficient staffing is closely linked to perceptions of job stress and burnout as well.

Limited cognitive resources. Cognitive human characteristics include information processing and decision making, knowledge and expertise, and human error. Humans have limitations of attention capacity, decision-making heuristics, and limitations to short- and long-term memory. These characteristics are important to consider when designing processes, devices, and even training programs and materials. Slips and mistakes are related to two different cognitive processes (i.e., automated mechanisms and higher cognitive and decision-making processes).

SUMMARY

Recurring evidence has shown that a large number of patients suffer injuries as a result of treatment, and most of the iatrogenic injuries are the result of errors. Two basic types of medical errors exist: human and system errors. Although human errors result from cognitive limitations, in many instances, the root cause of human error is poor system design. We can reduce human errors by understanding physical, cognitive, and psychosocial characteristics of people that establish our boundaries for safety. We can also understand the relationship of individual human performance to systems by understanding how individuals interact and are affected by workplace and organizational factors in the systems of care delivery in health. Human factors engineering is the study of factors and the development of tools that facilitate the improvement of human interaction with systems. The goal is to make the human interaction with systems one that reduces error, increases productivity, and enhances safety and reliability. An understanding of the inherent nature of errors and how human factors engineering relates is needed in order for us to develop appropriate strategies to improve human performance and the systems we function in to optimize safety in our healthcare environments.

A CLOSING CASE

Read the following case and use the questions that follow to apply what you have learned in this chapter:

While I worked as a dental assistant, I learned a lot about what goes on "behind the scenes" in a dental office. I do not think this office was unusual. There was drama, frustration, and a lot of work that needed to get done. Most of us had multiple duties every day. For example, the manager might double as an assistant if we were in a bind, or an assistant might take over the managerial duties and have to order supplies. Temporary employees, both dentists and assistants, were called in all the time, and some sort of change always seemed to be being made to the organization of the office.

One day, all of this confusion almost led to a mistake. A patient came in with high blood pressure, which is not unusual for people who are about to have numerous procedures done. Although she was on medication, her blood pressure was still very high; thus, we decided to give her some time to calm down. I told her that we were going to wait a little while until her blood pressure went down. I brought her a magazine and told her I would be back. When I rechecked it in 15 minutes, it was still high. At this point, the dentist spoke with the patient and asked whether she wanted to continue to wait or reschedule her appointment for another day. The patient chose to wait, so we obliged.

During the next hour, the entire staff had to hurry a little more because we had the same number of patients scheduled but one less room to treat them in because of the waiting patient. We were in overdrive mode when we returned to this particular patient. Usually, when a patient is at risk for any type of cardiovascular episode, we use an anesthetic without epinephrine. The dentist asked her assistant to prepare the anesthetic, but the assistant got caught up with another patient who had wandered out of his room. To be helpful, the dentist prepared the injection herself. She did not know, however, that she selected one with epinephrine. A few days earlier, the anesthetic had been ordered from a different company that color coded its vials differently. Usually, the green and red vials were anesthetic with epinephrine, and the blue were without epinephrine. The new company made blue vials with epinephrine. No one had informed the dentist because it was usually the assistants who prepared the injections.

The dentist returned to the treatment room and was about to inject the anesthetic when the assistant walked in with her prepared injection. She saw that the dentist had the wrong colored vial, immediately realized the mistake, and simply said, "Doctor, we have an emergency situation and we need your help." Of course, the dentist left the room without administering the anesthetic. The assistant walked into the dentist's private office where no one would overhear and explained the situation. The dentist returned to the patient, explained there wasn't an emergency after all, and gave the correct injection.

What would have happened if this patient had received the wrong anesthetic? She was having extensive work done, including extractions, and would have been given several injections at once before we had started doing anything. Fortunately, we never found out.

1. Describe the contributing factors to the system error in this case.
2. What human factors contributed to the error?
3. What changes would you suggest to make this office a "high-reliability organization?"

Discussion Questions to Launch Further Investigation

For further investigation, seek answers to these questions:

1. Distinguish between a slip and a mistake.
2. How does differentiating between these two types of errors help us in redesigning systems of care to improve patient safety?
3. Think about your own professional discipline. What are some of the responsibilities you have that match the skill-, rule-, and knowledge-based performance attributes?
4. What implications does the understanding of skill-, rule-, and knowledge-based performance levels have for learning and training in your profession?

REFERENCES

1. Schimmel EM. The hazards of hospitalization. *Ann Intern Med* 1964;60:100–110.
2. Steel K, Gertman PM, Crescenzi C, Anderson J. Iatrogenic illness on a general medical service at a university hospital. *N Engl J Med* 1981;304:638–642.
3. Bedell SE, Deitz DC, Leeman D, Delbanco TL. Incidence and characteristics of preventable iatrogenic cardiac arrests. *JAMA* 1991;265:2815–2820.
4. Brennan TA, Leape LL, Laird NM, et al. Incidence of adverse events and negligence in hospitalized patients: results of the Harvard Medical Practice Study I. *N Engl J Med* 1991;324:370–376.
5. Leape LL, Brennan TA, Laird NM, et al. The nature of adverse events in hospitalized patients: results of the Harvard Medical Practice Study II. *N Engl J Med* 1991; 324:377–384.
6. Bates DW, Gawande AA. Error in medicine: what have we learned? *Ann Intern Med* 2000;132:763–767.
7. Leape LL. Error in medicine. *JAMA* 1994; 272:1851–1857.
8. Kohn LT, Corrigan JM, Donaldson MS, eds. *To Err Is Human: Building a Safer Health System.* Washington, DC: National Academy Press; 2000.

9. Carayon P. *Handbook of Human Factors and Ergonomics in Health Care and Patient Safety*. Hillsdale, NJ: Lawrence Erlbaum Associates; 2006.

10. Reason J. *Human Error*. Cambridge: Cambridge University Press; 1990.

11. Hackbarth GM. Report to the Congress: Medicare Payment Policy. Available at: http://www.medpac.gov/documents/Mar09_March%20report%20testimony_WM%20FINAL.pdf. Accessed March 29, 2009.

12. Zhan C, Miller MR. Excess length of stay, charges, and mortality attributable to medical injuries during hospitalization. *JAMA* 2003; 290:1868–1874.

13. Donchin Y, Gopher D, Olin M, et al. A look into the nature and causes of human errors in the intensive care unit. *Crit Care Med* 1995;23(2):294–300.

14. Reason J, Hobbs A. *Managing Maintenance Error: A Practical Guide*. Burlington, VT: Ashgate Publishing Company; 2003.

15. Rasmussen J. Human errors: a taxonomy for describing human malfunction in industrial installations. *J Occup Accid* 1982;4:311–335.

CHAPTER 8

What to Do When Things Go Wrong

Linda S. Scheirton, Keli Mu, and Catherine Mahern

PURPOSE

The purpose of this chapter is to understand what to do when patient safety problems occur. The roles and responsibilities of healthcare practitioners, employers and healthcare organizations, and patients are described. The complexities of the interface between the "blame-free culture" and the concepts of accountability are explored. Ethical precepts of error disclosure, apology, and reparation are discussed.

OBJECTIVES

After completing this chapter, you will be able to:
- Describe "best practices" for the disclosure of practice error
- Describe the role of the legal system in patient safety and the duties arising under the legal system
- Discuss the role of peer review and the protections afforded to individuals involved in this process
- Compare and contrast healthcare's perfectibility model and "error-free" culture as opposed to the new view of a "just" culture
- Describe the process of "whistleblowing" and its impact on the individual(s) and institution
- Discuss the concept of moral management of error and the obligations that are associated with it

VIGNETTE

A family of four was driving home from an afternoon sporting event. The sky was overcast, and a severe thunderstorm ensued. The heavy rain caused low visibility. At a curve in the road, the automobile hydroplaned across the water, slid into a ditch, and hit a tall cedar wood fence at a wildlife refuge. The parents, who were in the front seat, had only a few cuts and bruises. The children, Isabelle, age 10, and Frédérique, age 7, had more extensive injuries. Isabelle had a right wrist fracture and a pneumothorax. Frédérique, who was sitting in the back seat on the right side, was struck in the face and mouth when the automobile hit the cedar wood fence. Both children were helicopter evacuated to the local medical center hospital. The mother was a psychiatrist, and the father was a local attorney. Several days after discharge, an outside orthopedist discovered that Isabelle's left arm was also fractured. The pain that she experienced while in the hospital had been attributed to the IV. When the pediatric surgeon learned of the misdiagnosis, he immediately contacted the family and apologized at length. The parents did not sue.

Frédérique, however, experienced severe mouth pain when in the hospital, and this continued after discharge. Her parents took her to see a local dentist, who diagnosed infection secondary to residual wood splinters. The family called and left a message with the answering service for the operating oral surgeon and resident. They did not receive a return telephone call from either doctor. The family then contacted the oral surgeon a second time but decided to speak with the hospital patient representative as well. They still did not receive a call from the oral surgeon. The parents decided to write a letter to the hospital chief of staff and one other system administrator. Immediately thereafter they received a letter from the oral surgeon stating that he was sorry that "Frédérique had such a difficult time with her injuries." Outraged at the unwillingness of the oral surgeon or resident to take even partial responsibility for the error, the parents sued. The case was settled out of court.

Although many errors are the direct result of individual failure, most errors are caused by system problems. Multiple errors that occur together usually cause the systems to fail. Health care is now transitioning from an old view of blaming, sanctioning, or firing to root cause analysis, learning from these errors and developing error-prevention strategies to promote patient safety. Along with that initiative is the practitioner's duty to disclose and report errors when they occur. The ethical rational for disclosure, based on the principle of autonomy, goes beyond what the law might require one to do. Patients have the right to be respected as persons and not to be deceived but to be fully informed instead. Nondisclosure undermines the public trust in the healthcare profession. Thus, truthful, timely disclosure of errors to patients is the obligation of all practitioners. To do otherwise constitutes a breach in professional ethics. It may also cause further harm or injury to a patient, those involved, and others. Nondisclosure of error undermines efforts to improve patient safety when practitioners are not enabled to learn from the errors of others. Likewise, patients must be informed about the inevitability of errors by their healthcare professional so that patients will adopt more realistic expectations. The moral management of error disclosure, reporting and knowledge of legal ramifications, and risk management must be operationalized and become second nature to healthcare practitioners.

BEST PRACTICES FOR ERROR DISCLOSURE

What Counts as an Error: How Do You Define or Distinguish It?

As noted in previous chapters, many error definitions are cited in literature.[1–7] According to a book on sentinel events by the Joint Commission on Accreditation of Healthcare Organization (JCAHO),[8, p.3] the terminology for errors "is far from fixed." The terms *bad outcome, sentinel event, adverse event, mishap, mistake, and untoward incident* are all equivalent or similar in meaning to the word *error*. Errors can be subdivided into individual and system errors, sometimes referred to as latent errors. System errors "derive primarily from flaws inherent in the system of [healthcare] practice," and individual errors result from deficiencies in the healthcare practitioner's "own knowledge, skill or attentiveness."[3, p.770] Furthermore, error can occur through acts of commission or omission, that is, what we do or what we fail to do. The JCAHO defines a sentinel event as an "unexpected occurrence or variation involving death or serious physical or psychological injury, or the risk thereof."[8, p.3] An error can cause major and minor harm. A "near miss," sometimes called a "close call," is an error that has the potential to do harm but is intercepted before harm actually occurs. Considerable debate in the patient safety literature has led many practitioners to question the necessity to disclose near misses or minor errors even though patients indicate that they would still want to be informed of these types of errors.[4,9–11] Actually, JCAHO developed patient safety standards and mandated a requirement for the disclosure of unanticipated outcomes in 2001.[11] The standard, like many standards, is open to interpretation as "unanticipated outcomes" may be viewed in either a broad or a more narrow sense.[12] Practitioners, professional organizational policies/opinions, and patient views are all divided on this question of whether all errors, major or minor, should be disclosed.[5,11,13,14] As guidance, a strategy offered by Hebert and colleagues is to look at minor and major errors in terms of proportionality. The need to disclose an error to a patient "increases as the harm or risk of harm to the patient increases."[15, p.512]

Ethical Precepts, Frameworks, and Organizational Ethics' Statements to Consider When Addressing Error Disclosure

Ethics is about choice. As practitioners, we must be able to distinguish between right and wrong and make choices that give rise to significant good rather than bad. Ethical theories, principles, professional codes of ethics, ethical decision-making models, organizational or institutional guidelines, and procedures are all available to guide us. A number of values, virtues, and obligations as well as potential and real consequences support or discourage error disclosure by practitioners. For example, the moral philosophical theory, deontology, guides practitioners by emphasizing our morally binding duty, obligation, and responsibility to inform patients when an error has caused them harm.[16] The practitioner is respecting the patient's dignity and autonomy by not lying and by acting out of beneficence. Likewise, the practitioner is violating the principle of nonmaleficence ("do no harm") when an error causes harm and is purposely concealed from the patient. This purposeful concealment may cause even more avoidable harm and injury than it would have if the error had been disclosed initially. The fiduciary relationship is necessarily one of great reliance whereby one party trusts and depends on another. In such relationships, the parties have unequal power. When a practitioner and patient agree to form such a relationship, a covenant is made. Maintaining the trust between the patient and the practitioner then becomes vital to the diagnostic and therapeutic processes. The practitioner agrees to honor that trust to become the patient's advocate in all health-related matters. Promoting the patient's best interest in such cases would include maximizing patient benefits while minimizing patient harms. If an error was to occur and result in patient harm, it would be a violation of the fiduciary relationship not to disclose that error. It would also undermine the public's trust in healthcare professionals as a group and undermine efforts for the improving practice safety.[15]

Deciding not to disclose an error could occur under what is known as paternalistic benevolence. This is intentionally overriding a patient's known preferences by another person, whose justification is the goal of benefiting the patient. For example, lying, nondisclosure, and partial disclosure of error are all interventions that could come under the "ethics" heading of paternalistic benevolence or the "legal" doctrine known as therapeutic privilege. Under the doctrine of therapeutic privilege, if disclosure would likely create an unreasonable risk of serious harm to the patient, the practitioner could invoke the privilege and not disclose the error. Examples of bad consequences of disclosure would be a physiologic response such as a heart attack or a psychological response such as an actual suicide or suicidal behavior. Antipaternalists argue that paternalism can never be justified because it restricts free choice. They will also point out that the therapeutic privilege violates the general moral rule of truth telling. It is certainly problematic to suspect that a practitioner can discharge the duty of a fiduciary while withholding information that bears substantially on the one person to whom the duty is owed; therefore, it would indeed be a rare situation to employ the doctrine of therapeutic privilege and justify such a moral departure.

Truthfulness is guided by two commands: "Do not lie" and "communicate with those that have a right to know the truth." Telling the truth can be difficult when it involves some personal risk such as fear of embarrassment or sanction, and yet it is an essential component of the practitioner–patient relationship. The virtue of truthfulness supports error disclosure to patients by practitioners. Truthful disclosure also allows the invoking of the principle of justice as fairness by allowing the patient to seek or accept reasonable restitution or recompense for harm done.

Guidelines and Mandates to Disclose Error

Most health practitioner codes of ethics such as the American Physical Therapy Association Code of Ethics, the American Nurses Association Code of Ethics, the American Pharmaceutical Association Code of Ethics, the American Occupational Therapy Association Code of Ethics, and the American Dental Association Principle of Ethics and Code of Profession Conduct all address issues of veracity, respect, trust, beneficence, nonmaleficence, justice, and fairness that would guide the practitioner in error disclosure. More specifically, the Occupational Therapy Code of Ethics, Principle 6.D. on veracity, indicates a therapist should "identify and fully disclose to all appropriate persons errors that compromise recipients' safety."[17] The American Medical Association Code of Medical Ethics standard relating to disclosure specifies that in situations where a patient suffers significant medical complications that may have resulted from a mistake, the physician is ethically required to inform the patient.[18] Other professional organizations have addressed this issue by developing policy statements on the disclosure of errors.[19] The organizational policy statement directs a physician to review carefully all relevant information when a human or system error has occurred. If the "physician determines that such an error has occurred in the care of a patient in the emergency department, he or she should provide information about the error and its consequences promptly in accordance with hospital policy on medical error disclosure."[19] One of the most influential organizations to develop patient safety-related standards for hospitals is the JCAHO, which adopted the standard in response to the Institute of Medicine (IOM) report published in 2000. The standard links disclosure of errors or adverse events to hospital accreditation. The pivotal standard requires "[t]he responsible licensed independent practitioner or his or her designee [to] clearly explain the outcomes of any treatments or procedures to the patient and, when appropriate, the family, whenever those outcomes differ significantly from the anticipated outcomes."[11] Even before the JCAHO requirements for disclosure were developed, one Veterans Affairs (VA) medical center had an active disclosure program[20] for more than 15 years, and the VA now has a program for all of its facilities.[21] In the VA's culture of accountability, it is required that an adverse event be disclosed to the patient, usually by "one or more members of the clinical team."[21, p.A-2] Royal Victoria Hospital in Montreal,[22] as well as the University of Illinois Medical Center, University of Michigan Health System, Kaiser Permanente, Catholic Health Initiatives, and COPIC Insurance Company,[23] are further examples of organizations that have had policies, procedures, or programs in place for disclosing error. A national study on hospital disclosure practices[5] indicates that approximately one in three hospitals had board-approved disclosure policies. The researchers attribute this number, as well as the substantial number of hospitals that are in the process of developing disclosure policies, to the reforms made as a result the IOM report, the JCAHO standard, and other safety initiatives. If the survey were administered today, the number of hospitals having disclosure policies would be substantially higher.

Statistical Facts, Barriers, and Benefits to Consider in Disclosure

Studies and reports cited in the literature suggest that disclosure does not occur as often as we would like. Wu and colleagues surveyed 254 house officers, and over half (54%) reported and discussed the errors with their attending physicians.[2] Only a small portion of the house officers (24%) disclosed the errors to the patients and their families. A survey of hospital disclosure practices found that disclosure occurred a mean of 7.4 times per 10,000 admissions. The researchers commented that "their study suggests that there is still a long way to go before serious harm is consistently and thoroughly disclosed to patients."[5, p.79] In a study by Martinez and Lo,[24] medical students reported witnessing significant errors but felt that many house staff and attending physicians were unwilling to appropriately disclose errors to patients. On the other hand, in a study involving focus groups, patients were unanimous in their desire to be told about any error that caused harm.[10] Results found in a vignette-based study revealed that 98% of the patients wanted some acknowledgment that the practitioner had made an error regardless of whether the error had caused harm to the patient.[9] Several grass-roots organizations such as Sorry Works! Coalition, Persons United Limiting Substandards and Errors, Consumers Advancing Patient Safety, and Medically Induced Trauma Support Services have been developed in an effort to advocate for disclosure of errors and apology. These organizations are raising awareness regarding patient safety and error reduction through advocacy, collaboration, education, and support.

An additional benefit of truthful disclosure of error may be lower liability payments for malpractice. One widely cited experience is the VA Medical Center in Lexington, Kentucky, whose disclosure policy and proactive stance on error disclosure have not resulted in higher liability as might be suspected.[20] Another study suggests that if patients' desire for honest and open acknowledgment of errors is honored, they may be less likely to sue.[9] Extreme honesty may be the best policy. Yet another benefit of practitioner disclosure is quality improvement. The American Medical Association Council on Ethical and Judicial Affairs' opinion entitled Ethical Responsibility to Study and Prevent Error and Harm, directs the physician to "offer a general explanation" to the patient "regarding the nature of the error and the measures being taken to prevent similar occurrences in the future."[25]

The discrepancy between disclosure practices that occur when errors are made by healthcare practitioners and the patients' preference for full disclosure is wide. A number of factors may help explain this discrepancy. The education of healthcare practitioners has been built around the perfectibility model. As students, teachers expect perfection, and as practitioners, patients expect it. Just as we strive for perfection, however, we must face imperfection. Disclosing errors brings imperfection to the forefront.

Fear can be a significant barrier to disclosure—fear of being labeled as incompetent, fear of legal repercussion, fear of creating patient anxiety, fear of a damaged reputation, fear of ostracism by peers, fear of loss of income, and fear for career advancement or retention. There may also be fear for the erosion of trust and respect between a practitioner and a patient when an error is made and then disclosed.

When a practitioner feels responsible for an error, he or she may experience persistent emotional distress such as shame, humiliation, remorse, devastation, inadequacy, and/or panic. The aftermath can be overwhelming for some and difficult at best for others. The practitioner should be encouraged to seek out a valued colleague in order to discuss the error and its personal and emotional impact. Giving emotional support to colleagues during times such as these will set the stage for future reciprocation and learning from the errors of others.

Responsibly communicating the error in an honest and empathic manner is also a positive step forward in clearing one's conscience. In the biblical sense, when one clears a conscience, there needs to be (1) self-acknowledgment, (2) a desire to acknowledge a problem, (3) an admission, (4) a feeling of regret (repentance) and accompanying apology, (5) restitution, and (6) accountability. Clearing one's conscience gives one the freedom to continue to serve whether that service is to God or to one's individual patient. This process can be very cathartic as well as emotionally and spiritually healing.

Can There Be a Just and Yet Blame-Free Culture?

Yes and no. Error "disclosure and accountability rest with both the system and the individual" practitioner.[26, p.65] Although individual performance and professional competence are extremely important, a practitioner may still make a number of errors because of conditions present that lie dormant in complex systems until activated by a series of triggering events. As we know, the genesis of error is multifaceted. Dysfunctional organization structure, inadequate training, poor design of equipment, faulty maintenance, and faulty communication all contribute to error-producing or latent errors. Errors can occur from ineffective, improperly designed, or flawed systems. In situations involving system error, it would be unjust to simply require the last treating practitioner to be fully accountable, accept blame, and disclose the error to the patient on his or her own. Blaming and sanctioning in this situation would encourage practitioners to hide their mistakes and avoid disclosure and reporting. It is a misconception to think that sanctions will lead to improved performance in the individual practitioner and at the same time act as a deterrent to error. Rather, blaming and sanctioning create a culture of fear, defensiveness, and often concealment that diminishes both learning and quality improvement. Instead, a nonpunitive culture should be fostered where practitioners are encouraged to disclose errors to patients and report errors through established mechanisms in order that quality improvement and error reduction occur. To do this, we must not view systems and individuals as adversaries or view punitive culture and blame-free culture as opposite ends of a continuum. A balance must exist between punitive action being taken for intentional violation of safe practice standards or reckless conduct on the one hand and an unintentional, inadvertent action on the other hand. A just system will require accountability when an action results in patient harm. A just system will examine how systems contribute to error. A just system will move away from blaming, sanctioning, and firing. A just system will call for a new systems-oriented ethical paradigm.[27] A just system will ultimately create an environment where practitioners are encouraged and supported for promoting safety, reporting errors, and disclosing errors to patients.

Best Practices When Things Go Wrong

Clear policies and procedures are paramount to fostering an institutional response to reducing errors and promoting patient safety. Full-disclosure programs such as those practiced at Veterans Health Administration, the University of Illinois Medical Center, and the Kaiser Permanente have been models for others to follow in the management of errors or adverse events. Sorry Works!, an advocacy organization for disclosure, apology, and upfront compensation after adverse medical events, recommends the development of a platform or an organizational infrastructure to support effective communication, coordination, and collaboration between healthcare professions, the patients, and their families.[28] The main purpose of developing a disclosure platform is to provide a standardized and consistent communication process for direction and support for all involved. Policy development, documentation, education, and quality improvement are all part of this platform.

These are suggested processes to follow when anticipating disclosure of error:

1. Decide what needs to be done immediately. The initial primary concern should be for the patient. Ensure that the patient is safe and "that an appropriate treatment plan is formulated and in place."[28, p.29] Take corrective action immediately, if indicated. A rapid investigation team should be readily available to determine what is known, the nature, and the circumstances of the accident. If possible, try to determine whether it is an authentic error. If it is an error, if known, determine the proximal cause. Define the known consequences, or potential or anticipated consequences, for the patient.

2. Decide whether to disclose. Most codes, disclosure policies, and professional guidelines are less clear on the level of error magnitude necessary for disclosure. In such cases, the proportionality rule may be invoked; that is, the need for disclosure "increases as the harm or risk of harm to the patient

increases."[15, p.512] Another strategy is to put yourself in the patient's position to determine how he or she would want the situation to be handled.
Cantor suggests systematizing the process of disclosure because it builds
consensus about whether disclosure is necessary.[29] For example, he believes
that both the practitioner and the organization should bear the responsibility for the disclosure process.

3. Decide when errors should be disclosed. Prompt timing for disclosure is
   important; typically within 24 hours of discovery is a good rule of thumb.
   Errors that require immediate healthcare interventions should be disclosed
   as soon as possible to avoid further patient harm. When uncertainties
   arise regarding the need for disclosure, consult with colleagues and supervisors for guidance or clarification. Providing timely, clear, and concise information to patients is imperative. Evasiveness, stonewalling, half-truths,
   or an outright unwillingness to answer questions may increase the chance
   for eliciting patient anger, anxiety, or suspicion. This can lead patients to
   mistrust the practitioner and the institution. Likewise, provide clear information regarding the plan for and management of an ongoing investigation to review what happened.

4. Decide who should be the most appropriate person(s) to disclose an error(s).
   According to the JCAHO, the person who must make the disclosure should
   be "the responsible licensed independent practitioner or his or her designee."[11, supra note 2] In certain situations, however, it could be deemed appropriate to have someone else on the healthcare team disclose if he or she
   is more knowledgeable about the error that just occurred. It is also prudent
   to have at least one other practitioner or administrator present during the
   disclosure process. Others recommend disclosure teams,[26] which are comprised of "high level" institutional representatives, the hospital risk manager,
   or quality control representative, for example. Liang does not think the
   practitioner should initially participate as a member of the disclosure team
   because the emotional stress generated from the error will potentially result
   in ineffective communication or conflict. The most effective person to use
   in such challenging situations is a level-headed person who can disclose the
   error objectively in a calm, nonreactive, caring, and honest way. The response to questions should demonstrate thorough knowledge of the event
   and be delivered in an accurate, nondefensive, and empathetic way. If no
   policy is available to guide the practitioner, each event should be evaluated
   individually to determine which level of direct involvement in the disclosure
   process is most appropriate. Ideally, those practitioners who participate

should be trained in the proper methods of error disclosure—the do's and don'ts of the disclosure process. The institution should invest in educational programs to heighten practitioner awareness and allow the opportunity to practice newly acquired disclosure skills. Gallagher and colleagues also suggest an improvement support system that provides "just-in-time" coaching so the coach can assist as the error event is unfolding.[30]

5. Decide to whom the disclosure will be communicated. Disclosure should be made directly to the patient, his or her family, or an official representative of the patient. If the patient is a minor or is incompetent, disclose to a family member or surrogate. It is suggested that patients be asked to bring along a support person (such as friend, family member, or significant other) to the initial disclosure meeting and any subsequent meetings. It would also be beneficial for a social worker, chaplain, psychologist, or patient advocate to be available to help the patient or his or her representative cope with the news.

6. Decide what components should be included in the disclosure. An honest and compassionate explanation about the error should occur within a reasonable length of time after the patient harm occurs or is discovered. Timing is important. Optimal timing of disclosure varies with the circumstances of error. Although there is the suggested 24-hour maximum disclosure rule, factors such as physical stability or time period between death and disclosure should also be considered. If a patient has expired, it is best to discuss the errors as soon as an initial investigation has occurred so that a more thorough explanation can be provided.[31] As previously mentioned, a rapid initial investigation could occur within a few hours and a meeting scheduled shortly thereafter. The explanation should include the circumstances, time, place, proximate cause of the error, if known, and the assurance that continued diligence will be used to discover the facts and analyze the error. In addition, it is important to let the patient know that the organization is committed to reducing the chances that another person will be harmed in a similar way.

   a. An open and forthright apology should be offered to the patient or family. A proper apology can be a powerful vehicle for fostering further open discussion; however, the type of apology that you decide to convey can have far-reaching tripartite implications from the ethical, legal, and religious perspectives. Liebman and Hyman classify apology in two ways.[32] First there is an "apology of sympathy" and second an "apology of responsibility." When a practitioner or disclosure team member offers an apology of sympathy, he or she is actually saying, "I'm sorry this happened to you." In contrast, if a practitioner or disclosure team member offers an apology of responsibility, he or she is actually saying, "I'm sorry we did this to you."[32, p.27] The apology of sympathy is often preferred by risk managers because there is no explicit admission of guilt and hence less of a legal risk. From a moral standpoint, however, an apology of responsibility is preferred when the practitioner is indeed responsible. In any event, a recent study by Mazor and colleagues[14] suggests that an apology of responsibility followed by full disclosure may cause patients to continue to trust their physicians and be less likely to change physicians when an error occurs. After all, we know that an apology of responsibility is in alignment with most professional codes of ethics. The assumption of responsibility and accountability by the practitioner is a religious imperative as well; therefore, disclosure and an apology, if done correctly, will act as the opening dialogue to repair the relationship between the patient and the healthcare practitioner and will hopefully lead to a negotiated agreement on reparations as well.

    b. Information should be provided regarding who will be managing the ongoing investigation and communicating up-to-date information back to the patient, family, or surrogate. This information should include the name(s) of contact person(s), their phone numbers, and their addresses.

    c. Provide the name(s) of practitioners who will manage the ongoing care of the patient and, if desired, offer to transfer the care to other healthcare providers.

    d. When indicated, an offer of recompense and/or arrangements for patient costs related to the error should be extended.

    e. Provide the patient, family, or surrogate with names of those who can continue to provide social, emotional, or spiritual help, if they desire.

7. Determine what is necessary for proper documentation. Memories fade quickly. When an error occurs, record the facts in the patient's chart in a timely manner. Also document what was disclosed to the patient, who said it, names, dates, times, and the outcome(s).

8. Offer support to the practitioner. The making of practice errors can lead to tremendous emotional distress. The practitioner may need to deal with feelings of guilt and self-doubt. Offering empathetic support mechanisms is humane, will hopefully make the healing process less difficult, and will facilitate future disclosure. After all, to err is human!

Special Aspects of Health Professional Student Disclosure

Health professional students should not initiate independent disclosure but may request to accompany the supervisor when communicating an error that he or she made by either omission or commission. Similarly, students may observe an error made by a clinical instructor, preceptor, or fieldwork supervisor. This can be awkward and confusing to students. They do not want to be put in the position of a whistleblower. Students have less training, experience, and adeptness in dealing with the complexities because of and as a result of their own error or errors of the healthcare professionals with whom they work.[33,34] Students may find it intellectually and emotionally challenging to explain adequately what occurred; therefore, students will not be expected to independently disclose to the patient. Even though there will always be a certain amount of uneasiness in these situations, it will be necessary, obligatory, and often mandatory to file incident reports for certain errors. Fortunately, established disclosure mechanisms are available to guide the student. Learning opportunities can occur through participation in morning reports, in-service sessions, consultation with the institutional ethics committee, grand rounds, mortality/morbidity conferences, and meetings with risk managers. Thus, a student can learn firsthand how to manage individual and system errors in health care and proactively contribute to an environment and culture of open disclosure and learning from errors made by others. Being confronted with these difficult issues early in a novice's professional career will serve him or her well in the management of similar situations in the future.

Final Analysis

When we review the myriad of ethical methods available to assist us in making decisions regarding disclosure of errors, the question still remains as to what should ultimately happen when we must distinguish between the right action and all other relevant moral aspects of ethics. Other moral aspects would include feelings, character virtues, and the impact of the action on ourselves and others (the consequences). Disclosing errors is emotionally and intellectually taxing. William Frankena, the author of the contemporary book *Ethics*, reminds us that "the only question we need to answer is whether what is proposed is right or wrong; not what will happen to us, what people will think of us, or how we feel about what has happened."[35, p.2] He insists that principles are the basic aspect of morality and that the other considerations such as "what will happen to me" are to be secondary. The generalized practice of open discussion and disclosure of practice errors will lead to better patient outcomes, improved professional morale, improved healthcare outcomes, a more realistic view of health care and what it can accomplish, and the possibility of fewer lawsuits and lower liability payments. In the end, moral management of error must become second nature to health practitioners in reducing errors and improving the health of the public.

REPORTING ERRORS

Reporting errors committed is the first step to learn from errors. Only by publicizing the adverse events are others able to understand the circumstances in which errors occurred, learn from the experience, and prevent similar errors in the future. The two primary purposes that reporting systems serve are holding healthcare practitioners accountable and improving patient safety.[36] Hence, professional organizations such as *American Society of Health-System Pharmacists*[37] and *Oncology Nursing Society,*[38] administrators, researchers, and practitioners in healthcare professions also strongly support and advocate for the development of error-reporting mechanisms.

In the IOM's report *To Err Is Human,* the recommended four-part plan to reduce errors in health care includes establishing error-reporting systems, specifically a mechanism to report errors to a body outside the healthcare organizations.[4] In the IOM report, the authors recommended two error-reporting systems: a mandatory reporting system designed to report errors that result in serious injuries or death and a voluntary reporting system intended to report less serious adverse event and near misses.[4] The mandatory reporting system is aimed at holding practitioners accountable, whereas the voluntary reporting system is focused on improving patient safety. The IOM report also asserts that it is each state's responsibility to establish a mandatory error-reporting system that is usually operated by a state regulatory agency. Voluntary reporting systems need to be fostered in healthcare organizations as well. The IOM report has become a catalyst for federal government, healthcare administrators, researchers, and practitioners to study mandatory and voluntary reporting systems to reduce errors and improve patient safety. To further the recommendations of this study, federal legislation has been enacted that will create a network of patient safety databases to be used to analyze national and regional reported information in an effort to identify error trends.[39] The U.S. Department of Health and Human Services is developing proposed regulations to implement the act. The plan is to create Patient Safety Organizations to collect, aggregate, and analyze information voluntarily reported.[40] After systemic and root causes of risk are identified, feedback will be provided to healthcare practitioners in an attempt to improve patient safety and quality.

The significance of error-reporting systems in improving patient safety cannot be overstated. Aspden and colleagues summarize the merits of error reporting as follows[41, p. 250]:

> Patient safety performance data may be used in support of many efforts aimed at improving patient safety: regulators may use the data for accountability purposes such as licensure and certification programs; public and private purchasers may use the data to offer financial or other incentives to providers; consumers may use comparative safety performance data when choosing a provider; and clinicians may use the data when making referrals. Most important, patient safety data are a critical input to the efforts of providers to redesign care processes in ways that will make care safer for all patients.

Currently, several systems are available in the United States for healthcare practitioners to report medical errors, adverse events, or near misses. For example, the U.S. Food and Drug Administration (FDA) manages two nationwide reporting systems for healthcare practitioners. The Vaccine Adverse Event Reporting System (VAERS) is in place to capture any information pertaining to any adverse events following administration of a vaccine product. VAERS is a cooperative program between the FDA and the Centers for Disease Control and Prevention. Reports to VAERS can be submitted via preaddressed postage paid report forms or using photocopies of or downloading the form from the FDA or Centers for Disease Control and Prevention website.[42]

The other reporting system operated by the FDA is the MedWatch program. MedWatch's Safety Information and Adverse Event Reporting System serves healthcare practitioners and manufacturers, as well as the "medical product-using public."[43] MedWatch is mandatory for manufacturers and voluntary for practitioners. The focus of MedWatch is on unexpected and unusual events and on newly produced drugs and products such as prescription and over-the-counter drugs, nutritional products, and medical and radiation-emitting devices. Reports to MedWatch can be sent via paper, fax, or the Internet. One major limitation with MedWatch is its difficulty in data mining because the reporting forms are scanned into the MedWatch computer system.

The United States Pharmacopeia (USP), in cooperation with the Food and Drug Administration and the Institute for Safe Medication Practices, operates the Medication Errors Reporting Program (MERP). Although MERP started in 1991, the USP has actually operated the error-reporting program for healthcare practitioners since 1971.[44] The USP MERP program is a voluntary, confidential, and practitioner-based reporting system, and practitioners can report medication errors via paper, telephone (800-23-ERROR), and the Internet. Error reporting can be anonymous if the reporter desires. MERP collects information relative to both potential and actual medication errors, and information collected with the USP MERP program will be forwarded to FDA and the product manufacturers after it has been review and analyzed by MERP. When reporting errors, MERP recommends that the following information be included[45]:

1. Description of the error or preventable adverse drug reaction. What went wrong?
2. Was this an actual medication error (reached the patient), or you are expressing concern about a potential error or writing about an error that was discovered before it reached the patient?
3. Patient outcome.
4. Type of practice site (hospital, private office, retail pharmacy, drug company, long-term care facility, etc.).
5. The generic name (INN or official name) of all products involved.
6. The brand name of all products involved.
7. The dosage form, concentration or strength, etc.
8. How the error was discovered/intercepted.
9. Your recommendations for error prevention.

Detailed information regarding the MERP program can be found on the Institute for Safe Medication Practices website.[45]

MedMARx is yet another reporting program under the auspices of USP. MedMARx is a subscription-based, anonymous, confidential, and Internet-accessible reporting system in which individual hospitals can submit medication errors collected via any error-detection method. Individual hospitals can use MedMARx as an internal performance improvement tool, but information collected by MedMARx is also analyzed and shared at a national level. A total of 13 required data categories in the MedMARx systems and MEDMARX data fields can be categorized by the type(s) of error, the cause(s) of error, the contributing factor(s), and the product(s) associated with reported errors. MedMARx was initiated in 1998, and more than 50 hospitals participated in its first-year operation.[46] Detailed information about MedMARx can be also found on the USP website.[47]

The Patient Safety Reporting System, launched in 2002, is a learning program developed jointly by the VA and the National Aeronautics and Space Administration. The voluntary, nonpunitive reporting and learning system is known for its confidentiality procedures, report management, quality assurance, and databases that are used for safety information distribution. The VA provides patient safety information in targeted publications to practitioners such as newsletters, alerts, and advisories.[48]

Other national voluntary reporting programs exist in addition to those discussed previously. In addition to these external voluntary reporting systems, Nash has also called for establishing proprietary error-reporting systems: "I am betting on the future success of tracking medical error with a private sector solution geared to help the individual hospital tackle the systems nature of medical error."[49, p.2]

The significance of error-reporting systems has also been recognized by the international community. In the United Kingdom, the National Patient Safety Agency of the National Health System has developed the National Reporting and Learning System for anonymous reporting of patient safety errors and systems failures by health practitioners across England and Wales.[50] The reported confidential data are analyzed by the National Patient Safety Agency to identify national patient safety trends and priorities and to develop practical solutions. Through Patient Safety International, the Advanced Incident Management System (AIMS) is being used by "over 400 Australian hospitals, as well as at sites in South Africa, New Zealand, and the United States. AIMS captures adverse event and near miss information across acute care, community care, disability care, mental healthcare, and residential aged care (nursing homes)."[51]

Despite the desired merits and intentions, many issues exist related to mandatory and voluntary error-reporting systems. For example, only 20 of 50 U.S. states have mandatory reporting systems in place.[52] The types of errors mandated to be reported vary considerably from state to state. The only reportable error common to all state reporting systems is unanticipated death.[49] Many factors appear to contribute to this undesirable situation. Research has suggested that the primary barrier for implementing mandatory reporting systems is practitioners' fear of repercussions, punishment, or litigations. Mandatory reporting also appears to support the creation of blame and punish culture, and increase liability exposures due to discoverability and confidentiality issues.[53]

Outcomes of mandatory and voluntary reporting systems in preventing/reducing errors and improving patient safety have shown to be encouraging.[54-61] For instance, when MedMARx was first operated in 1998, only about 50 hospitals participated in the program; however, in 2002, over 600 hospitals participated. According to the USP—released data in year 2000, 41,296 errors were reported by 184 healthcare facilities.[46] Voluntary reporting systems can improve patient safety by alerting us about new hazards and how they can be removed, dissimilating information about new methods to prevent errors, revealing trends and hazards that require priority attention, and recommending best practices for all to follow based on a central analysis.[61]

Although the benefits of reporting systems have been demonstrated, one of the major ongoing discussions is whether reporting errors should be confidential or anonymous. Confidential reporting, on one hand, ensures the ability to conduct needed follow-up interviews and seek more information from those who were involved in the incident. On the other hand, reporters may not trust the confidential reporting system and fear that reporting information may be disclosed and shared, which may consequently lead to punishment and litigation.[36] With anonymous reporting, the identities of the reporters are protected. Important information about the specific incident, however, may be missed with anonymous reporting because reporters may provide only enough information for others to understand the incident. Moreover, anonymous reporting also loses the ability to contact a specific individual about a particular incident if further information is needed.[36]

THE LEGAL SYSTEM

In the forgoing part of this chapter, we have made an ardent appeal for truthful disclosure to patients and prompt reporting of errors or even near misses. Disclosure fulfills the patient's fundamental right to information and can rebuild patient trust in his or her healthcare practitioner as well as in the healthcare system in general. Prompt reporting is by far the most effective way of preventing similar errors from being committed by other practitioners; however, whenever an error occurs and harm is being done, the patient automatically acquires a legal right to seek compensation for damages (a so-called tort). Furthermore, one of the primary purposes of the law is to prevent (further) harm, particularly harm that results from malevolent or negligent behavior. We have already seen that these legal consequences tend to render individual practitioners as well as healthcare institutions hesitant to disclose and report, even though in many instances those fears of the law are unnecessary. It is therefore important that practitioners have a solid understanding of what exactly the legal consequences are of errors, disclosure, and reporting.

TORT LAW

Definition and Justification

The definition of "tort" is somewhat elusive and includes a variety of causes of actions in law. The common element in all torts is that someone has sustained injury or loss as the result of (1) an act or (2) the failure of another to act where the law has imposed a duty. Through the payment of damages, tort law provides an incentive to prevent future harm. For the healthcare professions, an increasing awareness of the legal issues of professional malpractice can promote the implementation of mechanisms to improve care to patients.[62]

The most common tort is the tort of negligence. Four elements of negligence exist: first, a duty owed by one to another; second, a breach of that duty; third, harm or loss; and fourth, a causal connection between the negligent conduct and the loss or harm suffered. In other words, negligence consists of acting other than as a reasonable person would do in the circumstances or failing to use that degree of care for the protection of another that an ordinarily reasonably careful and prudent person would use under like circumstances.[63]

More simply, professional negligence is the failure to exercise the degree of skill and care that is the standard of the professional community. The duty owed to a patient arises from the provider–patient relationship. The duty requires a provider to exercise a level of care to a patient that is the recognized standard of medical care in the community that would be exercised by the provider in the same specialty under similar circumstances.[64] To provide care below that level or to depart from that standard would be considered a breach of the provider's duty to the patient. In order to sustain a malpractice claim, the damages sustained by the patient must have been proximately caused by the provider's breach of the duty. The law's recognition of the standard of care recognizes the difference between the harm resulting from the inherent risk in a procedure or treatment, the harm resulting from error, and harms resulting from recklessness or outright wrongdoing. Virtually all procedures and treatments have risk. Risk means that there is the possibility of harm arising from the treatment or procedure.[65] Where errors are likely to occur, protocols must be developed to reduce the likelihood of error. Failure to observe a protocol for error reduction is a critical piece of evidence that can be used in malpractice claims.

A provider who knows of an error and fails to reveal the error to the patient may increase the damages awarded to a patient where the failure to reveal deprived the patient of a timely opportunity to treat the injury. Concealing the error only increases the chances that a judge or jury would find proximate cause for the injury and compensate the patient.[66]

Tort law is generally designed to vindicate social policy, and the law of medical liability is the longest standing system used by society for reducing medical error and resulting injury to patients.[67]

Damages in Tort

Damages awarded to a patient are intended to restore that person to the position that he or she would have been in had the patient not been harmed. Under the principles of corrective justice, when a medical provider's negligence causes harm to a patient, the system requires that the negligent provider pay the patient to restore the patient to his or her previous position[68]; however, sometimes the patient cannot be restored and will suffer permanent disability. Where it is impossible to physically restore a patient, the law provides for the payment of damages to the patient in an amount to compensate for current and future monetary losses, as well as for the pain and suffering sustained by the patient. Pain and suffering includes past, present, and future pain, both physical and psychological. This might include humiliation and shame, loss of enjoyment in life, and loss of dignity.

Damages may also be awarded to the family of the patient where members of the family have also suffered loss due to the provider's breach of the standard of care. The loss of consortium is among the claims made by family members who have suffered loss due to the negligent action of a provider. Consortium has been defined to include loss of love, companionship, affection, society, comfort, solace, sexual relations, and services.[69]

In addition to the compensatory damages described previously, an erring healthcare provider may also be required to pay punitive damages. These are fines levied for the purpose of punishing a defendant. They also act as a deterrent for the defendant, as well as for others engaged in similar conduct, from repeating the wrongful act.[70]

Burden of Proof

A plaintiff—generally the patient who has been the victim of the error—in a malpractice action has the burden of proving the case for malpractice. This requires the plaintiff to call on expert medical witnesses to establish the standard of care in the community as well as the causal connection between the breach of that standard and the injury to the patient. Often in malpractice cases there are multiple actors, and a plaintiff cannot be expected to prove which actor or actors caused the harm. In such a case, where a plaintiff proves that each actor engaged in some torturous conduct that exposed the plaintiff to a risk of physical harm and that the torturous conduct of one or more of them caused the plaintiff's injury, the burden of proof on factual causation is shifted to the defendants.[71] A plaintiff must prove not only the elements of malpractice, but must also present evidence to establish the damages suffered. Experts such as economists and statisticians may be used to establish economic loss, and physicians and psychologists may be used to establish pain and suffering associated with the injury sustained.

In law there are three standards of proof by which a plaintiff may be required to establish evidence in order to prevail: beyond a reasonable doubt, by clear and convincing evidence, and by a preponderance of evidence. Proof beyond a reasonable doubt is used in criminal cases. Proof by clear and convincing evidence is required in cases involving a substantial right, often a constitutional right, and requires evidence indicating that the thing to be proved is highly probable or reasonably certain.[72] In all other cases, including medical malpractice, a plaintiff needs only proof by a preponderance of evidence to support the elements of the claim. Preponderance of the evidence means the greater weight of the evidence and is not related to the number of witnesses testifying to a fact. Rather, it refers to evidence that is the most convincing that "though not sufficient to free the mind wholly from all reasonable doubt, is still sufficient to incline a fair and impartial mind to one side of the issue rather than the other."[72, p.1220] In a medical malpractice case, this means that a plaintiff must prove that it was more likely than not that the recognized standard of medical care in the community that would be exercised by providers in the same specialty under similar circumstances was not followed and that it was more likely than not that the defendant's departure from that standard in the treatment of the patient was the proximate cause of the injury.

Employment Relationships and Liability

As already discussed, most errors that occur in the world of health care are not the result of a single practitioner, let alone a single practitioner who was willfully negligent. Rather, errors most frequently result from the complexity of the system in which care is delivered with many people and factors contributing to the error; therefore, when an error occurs, this raises the question about who exactly is responsible for what. In answering that question, tort law will generally look at the relationship among the team members with specific attention to lines of authority and control.

Employer Liability

Under the doctrine of respondeat superior, or vicarious liability, an employer is liable for the acts of an employee if the employee was acting within the scope of employment. Under respondeat superior, the employee stands in the shoes of its employer. This rule is premised on the idea that the one who is in a position to exercise control over the performance of a task must exercise that control or bear the loss that results. For example, a hospital may be held responsible for erring

behavior by a nurse employed by the hospital. There are many reasons for imput-
ing an employee's actions to the employer, including that employers have a measure of control over the employee, the employer initiated the activity out of which
the tort arose, the employer selected and hired the employee, and the employer is
in the best position to compensate harmed persons. Surely the employer is in a
better position to prevent the wrongful acts of an employee than is the person that
the employee harmed. This approach provides employers with an incentive to
carefully select employees and exercise control over the conduct of the employees.

An employer has a duty to hire and retain competent employees. The law im-
poses liability on an employer for the actions of its servants or agents if the employer was negligent or reckless in giving improper or ambiguous orders or failing
to make proper regulations, in employing improper persons in work involving risk
of harm to others or in supervising the activity. In addition to being liable for employees, an employee can also be liable for permitting, or failing to prevent, negligent or other torturous conduct by persons on the employer's premises or with
instrumentalities under the employer's control, regardless of the relationship of
those persons to the employer[73]; therefore, there is a cause of action available
against an employer for the tortuous conduct of an employee where the employer
has been negligent in hiring, training, supervising, or retaining an employee.

The relationship between providers in a medical setting is often complex.
Complex systems provide many opportunities for error, particularly where many
individuals have responsibility for a limited part of the process. When should a
physician be liable for the negligence of other healthcare practitioners? Should it
include when a nurse gives an improper medication and a patient is harmed? Is a
physician responsible for the results when he or she acts on a physical therapist's
incomplete or faulty entries in a patient chart? Is a treating physician culpable
when relying on a pathologist's incorrect laboratory report in determining the
course of treatment if an injury occurs? Should a physician be liable when a
healthcare practitioner is bound by his or her own professional duty to the patient,
independent of the treating physician? In the complex world of healthcare team
interface and provision of care, the potential for error with negative consequences
is substantial.

Some jurisdictions have recognized the validity of holding healthcare practitioners independently liable for their own acts. In these cases, the courts have
found that a physician does not exercise control over other practitioners' decisions
regarding the manner in which they carry out their duties. Physicians routinely
rely on other practitioners to carry out a treatment plan for a patient. In *Swigerd
v. City of Ortonville*, the court stated that "[a] physician can spend only a short

time at the bedside of each patient and he must therefore leave the actual fulfillment of his prescribed treatment to others. . . . If this were not the accepted practice, no person of moderate means could afford to employ [a physician]."[74, p.343]

Although physicians routinely order tests, prescribe medications, order therapies, and request anesthesiologists to prepare a patient for surgery, a physician does not control another healthcare practitioner's conduct. Physicians rely on the skill and competence of other practitioners carrying out their own duties to the patient. The same is true for other members of the healthcare team, all of whom have to rely on the competence and diligence of their fellow team members.

Even in jurisdictions that recognize a physician's right to rely on another healthcare practitioner's actions, a physician could be liable for the actions of other practitioners where the physician negligently hired or supervised the practitioner or retained the practitioner on staff after gaining knowledge of that practitioner's propensity for error.[75]

Independent Contractors

An independent contractor is a person who performs services for another person or entity but who remains independent from that person or entity. The independent contractor generally maintains a separate identity from the employer and is paid to perform the services with the work to be performed at the contractor's discretion. In the situation involving the conduct of an independent contractor, the employer is not generally held liable for the actions of that independent contractor. The rationale supporting this rule is that an employer usually does not have the right to control the manner in which the work is performed, as the work is that of the independent contractor's enterprise. In this case, it is the independent contractor, rather than the employer, who is responsible for preventing and distributing the risk[76]; however, this general rule is riddled with exceptions, primarily related to the employer's negligence in selecting or supervising the contractor. The status of a person performing services for another is a question of fact and not merely a question of how the parties characterize the relationship.

In determining whether a person performing services for another is an employee or an independent contractor, the courts look at the degree to which the employer exercises control over that person. If the employer controls the time, place, and method of the work performed, the person performing those services is considered an employee, not an independent contractor. As such, the level of autonomy exercised by the party performing the work or delivering a service is the hallmark of the distinction between an employee and an independent contractor.[77]

An employer is not liable for the actions of an employee if the employee is not acting within the scope of his or her employment. The courts have broadly interpreted the course and scope of employment and have determined that any action that bears a reasonable relationship to the employment is within the course and scope of employment. Only more significant departures from the work authorized for an employee will relieve the employer from vicarious liability for the employee's actions.

An employer may be held liable where there is a foreseeable risk of harm to others unless precautions are taken and the employer has failed to exercise reasonable care in selecting a competent, experienced, and capable contractor to perform the work. Likewise, after an employer has reason to know that the contractor has engaged in reckless practices or has neglected to take adequate precautions to prevent harm to third persons, the employer's failure to remove the contractor may result in liability to injured third persons.[78]

Peer Review as a Mechanism to Improve Safety and the Legal Barriers to Effective Peer Review

Peer review is the process by which medical professionals investigate, evaluate, and review the quality of care of their colleagues to determine whether it complies with the standard of care. Peer review serves as a tool for the improvement in the quality of service and to reduce medical errors.[79] It is intended to create an environment that is safe and confidential for all of the participants. It is through candid and open discussion and analysis that healthcare practitioners can detect errors and devise protocols to eliminate them, thereby increasing patient safety.[80] In order to reduce errors successfully, everyone in health care must participate in the effort to report errors, to identify the sources of errors, and to establish protocols and practices that will reduce human errors. The peer-review process occurs in hospitals, clinics, managed care organizations, and other healthcare delivery settings. Peer-review committees generally consist of practitioners with the specialized knowledge that is necessary to make medical judgments.[81]

Fear of Reporting

Many barriers to reporting medical errors exist; prominent among them is the fear of a malpractice claim against the practitioner or the hospital. The fear that information provided through cooperation with the peer-review processes may become available to lawyers in a malpractice action creates a chilling effect on participation in peer review.[82] Healthcare providers have voiced concerns about exposure to legal liability when reporting errors is mandatory and confidentiality is not guaranteed.[83] Without the protection of confidentiality, many providers fear that the information gathered from cooperating doctors, nurses, and other healthcare practitioners in a peer-review assessment will be seized by a plaintiff's attorney through discovery and will be used against them.[83]

Legal Discovery

Discovery is the term for the legal process in which parties in litigation obtain information to assist them in preparing their case. The U.S. Supreme Court has long held that the public has "a right to every man's evidence."[84, p.331] Through the discovery process, a party can obtain records, documents, reports, photographs, film, or data compilations that are relevant or likely to lead to relevant information regarding the case before the court. A party may take the deposition of any person with knowledge of any matter before a court. A deposition is the questioning of a witness under oath, generally before a court reporter, and is used to establish the facts in the case. A deposition can also be used to impeach a witness who testifies in court in a manner that is contrary to statements made under oath at a deposition. Generally, any person or entity can be compelled to produce documents or evidence and testify at a deposition if the information sought appears reasonably calculated to lead to admissible evidence. A court can also compel a party claiming bodily injury or psychological damage to submit to physical or psychological examination by an expert selected by the opposing party.

The rules for discovery set forth the manner in which discovery can be conducted and assist the parties in obtaining the necessary facts to evaluate and resolve their dispute fully. The discovery rules accomplish this objective by reducing the possibility of surprise, thus avoiding the necessity of conducting a trial in the dark. Discovery aids every party by narrowing the issues that are truly in dispute. Discovery exposes the weaknesses and strengths of the case for both plaintiffs and defendants and, after all of the facts are known, may encourage settlement.[85]

Privileges

In some limited circumstances, the law protects certain communications from the discovery process, as well as bars them from introduction at trial. This protection is known as a privilege, and it frees a person from any compulsion to give evidence. The theory behind any privilege is that although the information sought could be quite relevant and helpful to a judge or jury in determining liability in a particular case, there is a greater good in protecting the information. The U.S. Supreme Court has held that privileges should not be "lightly created nor expansively construed, for they are in derogation of the truth."[86, p.710] For some privileges, there is an underlying policy to encourage desirable communications between persons in special relationships. Communications between a doctor and a patient, a lawyer and a client, a confessor and a penitent, and a husband and his wife all enjoy the protection of a legal privilege. Many privileges evolved in common law through the courts; other privileges have been adopted by state legislatures.[87]

Many courts have followed a utilitarian approach to determine the utility of granting a privilege in light of the importance of the truth-finding function of the court. The courts use four criteria to evaluate whether a privilege should be recognized. The first criterion is that the communications must originate in a confidence that they will not be disclosed. This means that the communication was made in anticipation that it would remain confidential. The second criterion holds that confidentiality must be essential to the satisfactory maintenance of the relationship between the parties. This anticipates that the relationship must be one that relies on confidentiality as being an essential part of the relationship. The third criterion states that the relationship of the parties must be one that, in the opinion of the community, ought to be zealously maintained and fostered. Finally, the injury to the relationship from disclosure of the communication must be greater than the benefit gained by a litigant.[88]

These privileges exist because of the special value of these communications and the relationship between the communicators. These relationships, by their very nature, require that one party can rely on the other to hold their communication in confidence. In recognizing a privilege, the courts recognize and value the social policy of protecting certain communications regardless of the impact it may have on discovering the truth. Without the knowledge that a doctor will keep a patient's communications confidential, appropriate treatment received by a patient would be in jeopardy. As a society, we have placed a high value on the open and honest communication that takes place between a wife and husband, a healthcare practitioner and patient, a lawyer and client, and a member of the clergy and a penitent. These communications are valued so greatly that even if a man has admitted some grave crime to his wife, lawyer, or confessor, those individuals cannot be compelled to testify against him.

The primary holder of a privilege is that person whose immediate interests are harmed if there is a disclosure of the communication. Where a privilege exists, there is the possibility that a person has waived an otherwise valid privilege.

An example of a waiver is when an individual has communicated in confidence within a protected relationship but then also communicates the information to another person with whom no protection exists. If a reasonably avoidable third party is present at the time a confidential communication is made between protected persons, that communication may lose its confidential status, and thus, the privilege is lost.

A privilege recognized by several courts a product's or event's liability context is the self-critical analysis privilege, which is of great importance for peer review to be successful. Some courts have found that the ultimate benefit to others from self-critical analysis of a product or event far outweighs any benefits from disclosure.[88] The earliest reported case to recognize the self-critical analysis privilege was a medical malpractice case in which the plaintiff attempted to discover the hospital minutes and reports of peer-review meetings, including records of the meeting in which the plaintiff's care was evaluated. The court found that there was "an overwhelming public interest in having those staff meetings held on a confidential basis so that the flow of ideas and advice can continue unimpeded."[89] Other courts have refused to recognize the self-critical analysis privilege without statutory authority.

In order to foster peer review, however, most states have passed some legislation that creates a privilege for any person or entity making a report or providing information to a peer-review committee that is established for the purpose of maintaining and providing a high level of medical care.[79] By granting a privilege to the communications in the peer-review process, the legislatures of the various states encourage open communication. Without the confidence of knowing that the information shared in the peer-review process would remain confidential, healthcare practitioners would be hesitant to participate in a free and candid discussion. Without these protections, the goal of improving the delivery of health care would be difficult to attain.

Because peer-review statutes are adopted separately in each state, there is no uniformity in the law, and in fact, these laws vary significantly in their scope. To add to the confusion, the courts in each state have the opportunity to determine the breadth of the privilege granted by peer-review statutes, leading to inconsistent results.[90]

The existence of a peer-review statute that grants a privilege to a person or entity participating in the peer-review process is not an absolute guarantee that a litigant cannot obtain that information. The assertion of a privilege has a negative impact on the truth-seeking process in litigation and is the exception to the proposition that every person must provide evidence regarding any facts inquired of by a litigant. As such, the courts are hesitant to create privileges over and above those created by common law or by statute and will narrowly interpret the privilege in favor of full disclosure.

A significant part of the information that plays a role in the peer-review process may nevertheless not be privileged. For example, this privilege does not protect information that had its original source outside of the peer-review process. Common information such as medical charts, administrative records, personnel records, occurrence reports, investigation reports, and reports from other committees are not protected from discovery, as they are records kept in the ordinary course of business.

In interpreting the extent of the peer-review privilege, the courts in some jurisdictions have found that a person participating in a peer-review process was free to waive the privilege and voluntarily testify about the confidential proceedings.[79] Allowing any participant to waive the privilege, however, undermines the very purpose of peer review. Hence, some states have a statutory provision that any disclosure by a member of the peer-review committee shall not constitute a waiver of the privilege.[79] This enables the peer-review committee to keep its deliberations confidential and unavailable to a litigant.

When a litigant seeks records that a defendant claims are nondiscoverable under the peer-review privilege, the litigant may ask a court to determine whether the information requested is, in fact, privileged. If the court determines the information sought is privileged, the court may next determine whether that privileged information is discoverable under some statutory exception. Some state statutes permit a court to order the release of peer-review information when the patient has waived any privilege and the court, after conducting a hearing on the matter, finds that there is good cause arising from extraordinary circumstances.[91]

With each state adopting its own peer-review statutes and the courts of each state interpreting the meaning and intent of the statute, the present state of peer review as an effective mechanism to improve patient safety is in question. Until healthcare practitioners are assured confidentiality in the peer-review process, it is unlikely that all will enthusiastically participate in identifying, discussing, and reporting medical errors.

Resolving or Avoiding Conflict Where Errors Occur

The relationship between a healthcare practitioner and a patient is one based on trust. Where an error has occurred, particularly where the error results in injury, the failure of a practitioner to disclose such error to the patient is a breach of the trust placed in the practitioner by the patient. In addition to fulfilling an ethical ideal, disclosure can preserve the trust of a patient, as well as provide a practitioner with the opportunity to correct the error where possible.

The literature on the effect of disclosure on litigation is filled with stories as well as scientific studies on the benefits of disclosure on reducing litigation and the size of settlements.[3,20,92,93] Patients want to know the facts when an injury has occurred as a result of medical error, and along with that, they seek an apology. Litigation is often initiated by an injured patient in order to get the answers that healthcare practitioners have failed to give. Healthcare practitioners, fearing litigation, often avoid the candid discussion with the injured patient. Because of this fear, practitioners may deny a patient that which a patient seeks most. Where there is a medical error, patients want disclosure of the error, an explanation of how and why the error occurred, assurances that the consequences of the error will be mitigated, and assurances that a reoccurrence will be prevented, along with emotional support and apology where appropriate.[10]

Expressions of Sympathy and Apology

Open and frank communication between a healthcare practitioner and a patient is essential for a healthy provider–patient relationship. Because practitioners are afraid of how their words to a patient may be later interpreted in a court, they may be inclined to say little or nothing; however, the majority of states have passed legislation that makes inadmissible as evidence any statements, writings, or benevolent gestures expressing sympathy relating to an injury.[28] The overwhelming majority of state statutes that shield expressions of sympathy do not include any protection for an admission of fault that is made with statements of sympathy.[94] The use of the term "I'm sorry" or a similar expression should not be viewed as an admission of responsibility or negligence, but should be viewed as an expression of sympathy. In contrast, an apology communicates responsibility for an offense that includes an expression of remorse for the harm caused.[95]

Although the majority of states have statutes that prevent statements of sympathy from being used in court, some dispute the value of an expression of sympathy that is devoid of any expression of responsibility where an error has occurred.[28,83,93] In one study on the effect of apology on settlement decisions, an apology increased the likelihood of settlement, whereas an expression of sympathy alone fared no better than no expression of sympathy.[93] The offender offering a full apology was seen as experiencing more regret and as being a more moral person who is likely to be more careful in the future; the participants in the study also had greater sympathy and less anger toward the offender.[93]

An open dialogue regarding errors that have occurred may reduce the likelihood of litigation and extraordinary damages.[96] How an apology should take place depends on the circumstances and the people involved. In any event, the decision to make an apology must be coupled with an appropriate plan for the disclosure of the error and the apology. For every situation, there is a right way and many wrong ways to apologize. Because each patient, practitioner, and injury is unique, apologies should be tailored to address the unique situation presented. As discussed previously, healthcare practitioners and hospitals must work with risk managers to create a plan for disclosure and apology. Who should make the disclosure and apology? To whom should it be made? When should it be made? What should be said?

Litigation is expensive, time consuming, and stressful for both the plaintiff and the defendant in a malpractice action. Disclosing an error to a patient need not result in the end of an otherwise productive and satisfactory provider–patient relationship. Promoting open communication between a practitioner and a patient in the event of an error may increase the level of trust a patient has with healthcare practitioners and may reduce litigation.[3]

WHISTLEBLOWING AND ITS IMPLICATIONS

As we have seen, an error is distinct from negligence. Negligence is the failure to perform at the level of competency consistent with professional norms of practice and operation where that failure leads to harm; however, a competent practitioner given the right circumstances can err. As part of a supportive, nonpunitive learning culture, these errors should be reported, analyzed, and disclosed, and improvements in patient safety should be made; however, instances exist where the healthcare practitioner can observe a fellow practitioner that exhibits reckless behaviors, intentionally violates procedural rules, is abusive or even negligent in caring for patients, or continues to disregard his or her own errors. In order to remove or prevent harm to patients, a practitioner may need to "blow the whistle" on a fellow practitioner. The term "whistleblower" originated in England from the bobbies' use of whistles to indicate a crime in progress.[97] In the area of employment, a whistleblower is a person who believes that public interest overrides the interests of the organization and publicly exposes the organization's conduct that is harmful to individuals or to the public. The purpose of whistleblowing is to stop the wrongdoing by an organization by exposing its conduct to the light. The implications of whistleblowing can be tremendous. Whistleblowers place their jobs, reputations, and careers on the line in order to protect the public. Although some whistleblowers are hailed as heroes, many are looked on with disdain and contempt.

On one hand, we would like to believe that an individual employee would expose an organization's misdeeds that could harm another; we also place a high value on loyalty within organizations. The whistleblower that goes forward to expose an organization's misdeeds is often perceived as a tattletale, squealer, traitor, rat, fink, or informer. Much of this stems from the sense that the employee has publicly harmed the very organization that provides the whistleblower's livelihood. These pejorative terms do not reflect the value of the positive outcomes that often result from a whistleblower's actions but instead reflect how some view a breach of loyalty.

Many people spend as much time, sometimes more, with co-workers than they spend with their families. At work, strong relationships are often formed, and a sense of loyalty is developed. Most people do not work in isolation but work in an environment where one person's productivity is dependent on many others, a team as it were; however, if employees work on a "team" and their supervisor is the coach, urging them on to success, where is the referee who will "blow the whistle" when the fundamental rules are broken? Within the professions, such as medicine, there is an elevated level of cohesion that may make whistleblowing less likely to occur. Although in medicine there is a high sense of loyalty to one's colleagues, loyalty to patients comes first.[98]

A not uncommon result of whistleblowing is retaliation in the workplace. Employers may retaliate by demoting, harassing, denying advancement, or firing in order to enforce employee loyalty, preserve morale, and preserve company security and procedures.[99] In addition to the possibility of being terminated from employment, a whistleblower's career may be in jeopardy. Other employers may not be interested in hiring a person who blew the whistle at a previous job. Most employees know the possible consequences from whistleblowing and are intimidated by the prospect of retaliation. Making the decision to blow the whistle on an organization can have an emotional toll on the employee. Even when not terminated from employment, the whistleblower may face both personal and professional isolation and may be placed in the position of a scapegoat.[98]

In spite of the risks associated with whistleblowing, a medical provider must acknowledge that the failure to report serious misconduct is to become an accessory to that conduct. Whistleblowing, although to be used as a last resort, provides an important gatekeeping function to the medical professions.

Of course, there is the potential for great benefits arising from whistleblowing. Primary among these is the elimination of wrongdoing. In the medical professions, whistleblowing can improve the quality of care for patients by promoting change in the organization. Additionally, the decision to blow the whistle can fulfill one's sense of ethical duty to patients as well as to the profession. In the case of a provider with alcohol or drug addiction, addressing the wrongful conduct can result in the provider obtaining the necessary assistance to overcome the addiction.

Before blowing the whistle, an employee should develop a strategy for action. It is important to try to settle the matter internally, and whistleblowing should be viewed as a last resort because of its destructive side effects. An employee who has concerns about a medical provider's conduct should engage in self-analysis to determine whether the conduct is merely different than what the employee would expect or whether it fails to meet the minimum standard of care and harm is likely to occur. If the self-analysis does not resolve the employee's concerns about the conduct, a written summary of the situation should be prepared and relevant facts documented. If possible, the employee should consult with other healthcare providers to validate the concern.

It is often best for an employee to discuss the concerns directly with the responsible provider by calling the conduct to the attention of the provider; however, approaching the wrongdoer may not always be easy in a setting where the employee is subordinate to the wrongdoer. By approaching the alleged wrongdoer and engaging in a dialogue about the issue, the employee may find that her concerns have been resolved.

If the employee has discussed the matter with the wrongdoer and no resulting positive change has occurred or the employee does not feel capable of discussing the matter directly with the wrongdoer, the employee should report the conduct to a supervisor. At this stage, documentation is extremely important, and the facts must not be exaggerated or embellished. The weight of the evidence gathered strengthens the report. A whistleblower is a witness, not a complainant, and the focus of the report must be on patient care and the factual nature of the conduct of the wrongdoer. A whistleblower must recognize the effects of speaking out and the possible harm to the person or the institution in doing so and make every effort to validate every fact before speaking out.[100]

If, after going to a supervisor, there has been no change in conduct or procedure, the employee may report the wrongdoing to those higher up in the organization, and only after doing so should an employee become a whistleblower and report the problem to an outside agency. The problem with this approach is that going through the previously mentioned steps can be very time consuming. If an immediate threat of harm to other patients exists, then an employee may feel that it is necessary to shorten the process. In following the multistep process, the organization has the opportunity to build a case against the whistleblower.

Historically, unless there was an agreement providing otherwise, most employees held their position at the will of the employer, and the employer had the right to discharge an employee for any, or for that matter, no reason[97,99]; however, through the adoption of legislation and the development of case law, it is now recognized that an employer may not discharge an employee because of discrimination based on race, gender, age, religion, and so forth. There is also some restriction on the discharge of whistleblowers.

The protection for whistleblowers has been slow and narrowly applied. The first case to provide a public policy exception to the employment-at-will doctrine was in *Peterman v. International Brotherhood of Teamsters*.[101] Peterman refused to follow his employer's request that he falsely testify to a legislative committee. Peterman was fired, and the employer argued that Peterman was an employee at-will and thus could be fired for any reason. The court disagreed and found that public policy dictates that one's continued employment should not be contingent on the commission of a felony at the insistence of an employer.

Although the majority of the courts recognize the public policy exception to the at-will employment doctrine, its application has been narrow in scope and has not been extended to solely safeguard private concerns such as an employee's conscience. The courts have been slow to extend the public policy exception to cover whistleblowers. Courts recognize the competing interests of employer discretion, employee security, and public policy.[97]

The majority of the states, as well as Congress, have passed legislation to protect the whistleblower,[99] but the laws leave significant gaps. Most states have enacted statutes that provide that private-sector employees cannot be terminated for blowing the whistle on issues of public health and safety. Many laws apply only to government whistleblowers or whistleblowers in certain industries.[102] Section 806 of the Sarbanes-Oxley Act[103] gave at-will employees in the private sector protection for disclosing malfeasance that affects the price of publicly traded companies, but this patchwork of laws, both federal and state, leaves many people vulnerable to retaliation for whistleblowing. Employees should not bear the brunt of responsibility for speaking out against their employers who engage in illegal or wrongful conduct. Only through whistleblower protection will employees have the tools to step up and fight for what is right without fear of retaliation, and employers will feel a sense of responsibility and accountability to the public.

There is also danger in false accusations being made by persons who are disappointed in their work, malicious toward their employer or co-worker, or incompetent and who rush to make public accusations.[100] False accusations result in a loss of trust that undermines the productivity of an organization. If an investigation ensues, the victim will experience an invasion of privacy and will likely sustain a loss of respect, even if cleared of the accusation. These malcontents undermine the courageous individuals who risk so much to honor their professional and personal codes of ethics. In spite of the negative consequences suffered from false accusations, society cannot risk silencing those who blow the whistle for legitimate reasons in the hope of eliminating false accusations.

Organizations can develop effective internal whistleblowing procedures that effectively address the concerns of employees as well as maintain the integrity and reputation of the organization. This can be accomplished by establishing an authority within the organization with the power to address issues raised, by encouraging employees to take their concerns to this authority, and by showing the employees that the organization is serious about addressing violations of any established code of conduct.[104] Employees must view this as a trustworthy process by subordinates and must be confident that whistleblowers will be protected from retaliation in the workplace.

SUMMARY

The practice of disclosing errors to patients is a positive movement toward a goal of transparency in health care. When a healthcare practitioner is honest, trust is maintained. Doing the "right" thing may even decrease the likelihood of lawsuits. Morally managing error has the enormous potential to improve patient-centered outcomes. Ultimately, a just culture can be created when practitioners are encouraged and supported for promoting safety, reporting errors, and disclosing errors to patients.

A CLOSING CASE

Read the following case and use the questions that follow to apply what you have learned in this chapter:

A third-year pharmacy student is employed as a pharmacy intern at a local neighborhood community pharmacy. While working at the cash register, a client approaches. The client is a professor in the pharmacy program in which the student is enrolled. The student recognizes the professor's face and cordially says hello.

The professor and pharmacy student engage in small talk about the pharmacy program at the university, and the professor tells the pharmacy student that she has come to pick up her prescription. The professor neither gives her name nor does the pharmacy student request her name. The pharmacy student walks to the "filled" prescription bins and hands her the prescription of another client. He proceeds to call her by the name "Anne." Her name is "Linda."

The pharmacy professor looks down at the label on the small white paper bag. She notices that the prescription label denotes a drug for which she has had a severe allergic reaction to in the past. It is not her name on the label but the name of a colleague that is employed at the same university with an office located just three doors down the hall from her own. She promptly tells the pharmacy student that she is not "Anne." The pharmacy student is quite embarrassed and immediately acknowledges that he mistook her for "Anne."

"I've had several university faculty and staff come in here today." He nervously laughs and says, "I know who you are! Here is 'your' prescription."

1. This is categorized as a wrong person, wrong site, and/or wrong procedure error. If you had been the pharmacy student that had committed the error, how would you have managed it?
2. Write a narrative of this case using moral management strategies and concepts found in this chapter. How could this same error be avoided in the future? What system changes would you put in place to ensure that this does not occur again?

REFERENCES

1. Leape LL. Error in medicine. *JAMA* 1994;272:1851–1857.
2. Wu AW, Folkman S, McPhee SJ, Lo B. Do house officers learn from their mistakes? *JAMA* 1991;265:2089–2094.
3. Wu AW, Cavanaugh TA, McPhee SJ, Lo B, Micco GP. To tell the truth: ethical and practical issues in disclosing medical mistakes to patients. *J Gen Intern Med* 1997;12:770–775.
4. Kohn LT, Corrigan JM, Donaldson MS, eds. *To Err is Human: Building a Safer Health System.* Washington, DC: National Academy Press; 2000.
5. Lamb RM, Studdert DM, Bohmer RMJ, Berwick DM, Brennan TA. Hospital disclosure practices: results of a national survey. *Health Aff* 2003;22:73–83.
6. Scheirton L, Mu K, Lohman H. Occupational therapists' responses to practice errors in physical rehabilitation settings. *Am J Occup Ther* 2003;57:307–314.
7. National Quality Forum. *Standardizing a Patient Safety Taxonomy: A Consensus Report.* Washington, DC: National Quality Forum; 2006.
8. Joint Commission on Accreditation of Healthcare Organizations. *Sentinel Events: Evaluating Cause and Planning Improvement,* 2nd ed. Oakbrook Terrace, IL: Joint Commission on Accreditation of Healthcare Organizations; 1998.
9. Witman AB, Park DM, Hardin SB. How do patients want physicians to handle mistakes? *Arch Intern Med* 1996;156:2565–2569.

10. Gallagher T, Waterman A, Ebers A, Fraser V, Levinson W. Patients' and physicians' attitudes regarding the disclosure of medical errors. *JAMA* 2003;289:1001–1007.
11. Joint Commission on Accreditation of Healthcare Organizations. Hospital Accreditation Standards RI.1.2.2. July 1, 2001.
12. LeGros N, Pinkall JD. The new JCAHO patient safety standards and the disclosure of unanticipated outcomes. *J Health Law* 2002;35:189–210.
13. Mazor KM, Simon SR, Yood RA, et al. Health plan members' views about disclosure of medical errors. *Ann Intern Med* 2004;140:409–418, E419–E423.
14. Mazor KM, Simon SR, Gurwitz JH. Communicating with patients about medical errors. *Arch Intern Med* 2004;164:1690–1697.
15. Hebert PC, Levin AV, Robertson G. Bioethics for clinicians: 23: disclosure of medical error. *Can Med Assoc J* 2001;164:509–513.
16. Bernstein M, Brown B. Doctors' duty to disclose error: a deontological or Kantian ethical analysis. *Can J Neurol Sci* 2004;31:169–174.
17. American Occupational Therapy Association. The occupational therapy code of ethics. *Am J Occup Ther* 2005;59:639–642.
18. American Medical Association. Code of Medical Ethics of the American Medical Association. Council on Ethical and Judicial Affairs. Current Opinions with Annotations. E-8.12 Patient information, Issued March 1981; Updated June 1994. Chicago, IL: American Medical Association; 2008.
19. American College of Emergency Physicians. Disclosure of Medical Errors. Available at: http://www.acep.org/practres.aspx?id=29178. Accessed March 31, 2009.
20. Kraman SS, Hamm G. Risk management: extreme honesty may be the best policy. *Ann Intern Med* 1999;131:963–967.
21. Veterans Health Administration. *Disclosure of Adverse Events to Patients*, VHA Directives 2008–002, Washington, DC: Department of Veterans Affairs; 2008.
22. Peterkin A. Guidelines covering disclosure of errors now in place at Montreal hospital. *Can Med Assoc J* 1990;142:984–985.
23. Shapiro, E. Disclosing Medical Errors: Best Practices from the "Leading Edge." Available at: www.arpatientsafety.com/. Accessed March 31, 2009.
24. Martinez W, Lo B. Medical students' experiences with medical errors: an analysis of medical student essays. *Med Educ* 2008;42:733–741.
25. American Medical Association. Code of Medical Ethics of the American Medical Association. Council on Ethical and Judicial Affairs. Current Opinions with Annotations. E-8.121 Ethical Responsibility to Study and Prevent Error and Harm, Adopted June 2003. Chicago, IL: American Medical Association; 2008.
26. Liang BA. A system of medical error disclosure. *Qual Saf Health Care* 2002;11:64–68.
27. Liang BA. A policy of system safety: shifting the medical and legal paradigms to effectively address error in medicine. *Harv Health Policy Rev* 2004;5:6–13.
28. Wojcieszak D, Saxton JW, Finkelstein MM. *Sorry Works! Disclosure, Apology, and Relationships Prevent Medical Malpractice Claims.* Bloomington, IN: AuthorHouse; 2008.
29. Cantor MD. Telling patients the truth: a systems approach to disclosing adverse events (medical error disclosure). *Qual Saf Health Care* 2002;11:7.
30. Gallagher T, Denham C, Leape L, Amori G, Levinson W. Disclosing unanticipated outcomes to patients: the art and practice. *J Patient Saf* 2007;3:158–165.
31. Selbst SM. The difficult duty of disclosing medical errors. *Contemp Pediatr Arch* 2003;20:51.
32. Liebman CB, Hyman CS. A mediation skills model to manage disclosure of errors and adverse events to patients. *Health Aff* 2004;23:22–32.

33. Crook ED, Stellini M, Levine D, Wiese W, Douglas S. Medical errors and the trainee: ethical concerns. *Am J Med Sci* 2004;327(1):33–37.
34. Wusthoff CJ. Medical mistakes and disclosure: the role of the medical student. *JAMA* 2001;286:1080–1081.
35. Frankena W. *Ethics.* Englewood Cliffs, NJ: Prentice Hall; 1963.
36. Beyea SC. Reporting medical errors and adverse events. *AORN J* 2002;75:853–855.
37. American Society of Health-System Pharmacists. ASHP statement on reporting medical errors. *Am J Health Syst Pharm* 2000;57:1531–1532.
38. Oncology Nursing Society. Oncology Nursing Society Position: Prevention and Reporting of Medication Errors. Available at: http://www.ons.org/publications/positions/documents/pdfs/MedicationErrors.pdf. Accessed March 31, 2009.
39. Patient Safety and Quality Improvement Act of 2005. Public Law 109-41, 42, U.S.C.
40. Physicians Want to Learn from Medical Mistakes but Say Current Error-Reporting Systems Are Inadequate [press release]. Rockville, MD: Agency for Healthcare Research and Quality; January 9, 2008. Available at: http://www.ahrq.gov/news/press/pr2008/errepsyspr.htm. Accessed March 31, 2009.
41. Aspden P, Corrigan JM, Wolcott J, Erickson SM. Patient safety reporting systems and applications. In: Aspden P, Corrigan JM, Wolcott J, Erickson SM, eds. *Patient Safety: Achieving a New Standard for Care.* Washington, DC: The National Academy Press.
42. U.S. Food and Drug Administration. Vaccine Adverse Event Report System. Available at: http://www.fda.gov/cber/vaers/vaers.htm. Accessed March 31, 2009.
43. U.S. Food and Drug Administration. MedWatch: The FDA Safety Information and Adverse Event Reporting System. Available at: http://www.fda.gov/medwatch/. Accessed March 31, 2009.
44. Cohen MR, ed. *Medication Errors.* Washington, DC: American Pharmaceutical Association; 1999.
45. Institute for Safe Medication Practices. ISMP Medication Errors Reporting Program (MERP). Available at: http://www.ismp.org/orderforms/reporterrortoISMP.asp. Accessed March 31, 2009.
46. Phillips MA. Voluntary reporting of medication errors. *Am J Health Syst Pharm* 2002;59:2326–2328.
47. U.S. Pharmacopeia MEDMARX©. Available at: http:www.usp.org/hqi/patientSafety/medmarx/. Accessed March 31, 2009.
48. Department of Veterans Affairs and the National Aeronautics and Space Administration. Patient Safety Reporting System. Available at: http://www.psrs.arc.nasa.gov. Accessed March 31, 2009.
49. Nash DB. Tracking medical errors: enter the private sector. *Health Policy News* 2003; 16:1–3.
50. National Patient Safety Agency. National Reporting and Learning System. Available at: http://www.npsa.nhs.uk/patientsafety/reporting. Accessed March 31, 2009.
51. Patient Safety International. Advanced Incident Management System (AIMS). Available at: http://www.patientsafetyint.com. Accessed March 31, 2009.
52. Simpson KR, Maher MA, Berry MC. Second opinion. Should there be mandatory reporting of medical errors? Writing for the pro position . . . writing for the con position. *Am J Matern Child Nurs* 2001;26:120–121.
53. Antonow JA, Smith AB, Silver MP. Medication error reporting: a survey of nursing staff. *J Nurs Care Qual* 2000;15:42–48.
54. Cousins DD. Developing a uniform reporting system for preventable adverse drug events. *Clin Ther* 1998;20:c45–c58.

55. Gawande AA, Zinner MJ, Studdert DM, Brenna TA. Analysis of errors reported by surgeons at three teaching hospitals. *Surgery* 2003;133:614–621.

56. Kobus DA, Amundson D, Moses JD, Rascona D, Gubler KD. A computerized medical incident reporting system for errors in the intensive care unit: Initial evaluation of interrater agreement. *Mil Med* 2001;166:350–353.

57. Osmon S, Harris CB, Dunagan WC, Prentice D, Fraser VJ, Kollef MH. Reporting of medical errors: an intensive care unit experience. *Crit Care Med* 2004;32:727–733.

58. Pace WD, Staton EW, Higgins GS, Main DS, West DR, Harris DM. Database design to ensure anonymous study of medical errors: a report from the ASIPS Collaborative. *JAMA* 2003;10:531–540.

59. Weingart SN, Callanan LD, Ship AN, Aronson MD. A physician-based voluntary reporting system for adverse events and medical errors. *J Gen Intern Med* 2001;16:809–814.

60. Meurier CE. Understanding the nature of errors in nursing: using a model to analyze critical incident reports of errors which had resulted in an adverse or potentially adverse event. *J Adv Nurs* 2000;32:202–207.

61. Leape LL. Reporting of adverse events. *N Engl J Med* 2002;347:1633–1638.

62. Ranke BA, Moriarty MP. An overview of professional liability in occupational therapy. *Am J Occup Ther* 1997;51:671–680.

63. 57A Am. Jur.2nd, Negligence § 225, 2008.

64. 65 C.J.S. Negligence § 164, 2008.

65. Shelton JD. The harm of "First Do No Harm." *JAMA* 2000;284:2687.

66. Kapp MB. Legal anxieties and medical mistakes: barriers and pretexts. *J Gen Intern Med* 1997;12:787–788.

67. Liang BA. The adverse event of unaddressed medical error: identifying and filling the holes in the health-care and legal systems. *J Law Med Ethics* 2001;29:346–368.

68. Brushwood DB, Mullan K. Corporate pharmacy's responsibility for a dispensing error. *Am J Health Syst Pharm* 1996;53:668–670.

69. Joslyn DR. Annotation. *Wife's right of action for loss of consortium.* 36 A.L.R.3d (1971).

70. Sunstein CR, Hastie R, Wayne JW, Schkade DA, Viscusi WK. *Punitive Damages: How Juries Decide.* Chicago, I: University of Chicago Press; 2002.

71. Restatement (Third) of Torts: Liability for Physical Harm § 28 (Draft No. 5, 2008).

72. *Black's Law Dictionary,* 8th ed. St. Paul, MN: West Publishing Company; 2004.

73. Restatement (Second) of Agency § 213 (1971).

74. *Swigerd v. City of Ortonville,* 246 Minn. 339, (Minn. Sup. Ct. 1956).

75. Lisk L. A physician's respondeat superior liability for the negligent acts of other medical professionals—when the captain goes down without the ship. *Univ Ark Little Rock Law J* 1991;13:183–207.

76. Richard G. Master and servant—liability for injury to third parties: employer's vicarious liability to employees of an independent contractor. *N D Law Rev* 1996;72:181–195.

77. Calvert Hanson L. Employers beware! Negligence in the selection of an independent contractor can subject you to legal liability. *Univ of Miami Bus Law J* 1995;5:129–155.

78. Keeton W, Dobbs D, Keeton R, Owen D, eds. *Prosser and Keeton on Torts,* 5th ed. Eagan, MN: West Group Publishers; 1984, pp. 509–514.

79. Kohlberg KR. The medical peer review privilege: a linchpin for patient safety measures. *Mass Law Rev* 2002;86:157–161.

80. Friend GN, Rangel JL, Finch M, Storm BA. The new rules of show and tell: identifying and protecting the peer review and medical committee privileges. *Bayl Law Rev* 1997;49:607–656.

81. Rodgers A. Procedural protections during medical peer review: a reinterpretation of the Health Care Quality Improvement Act of 1986. *Pa State Law Rev* 2007;111:1047.

82. Liang BA. Error in medicine: legal impediments to U.S. reform. *J Health Polit Policy Law* 1999;24:27–58.

83. Landsman S. Reflections on jury phobia and medical malpractice reform. *De Paul Law Rev* 2008;57:221–241.

84. *U.S. v. Bryan*, 339 U.S. 323 (1950).

85. 23 Am. Jur.2d, Depositions & Discovery § 1, 2008.

86. *U.S. v. Nixon*, 418 U.S. 683 (1974).

87. Weiner J. "And the wisdom to know the difference": confidentiality vs. privilege in the self-help setting. *Univ PA Law Rev* 1995;144:243–307.

88. *Bradley v. Melroe*, 141 F.R.D. 1 (D.D.C. 1992).

89. *Bredice v. Doctor's Hospital*, 50 F.R.D. 249 (D.D.C. 1970).

90. Nijm LM. Pitfalls of peer review: the limited protection of state and federal peer review law for physicians. *J Leg Med* 2003;24:541–556.

91. Liang BA. Promoting patient safety through reducing medical error: a paradigm of cooperation between patient, physician, and attorney. *South Ill Univ Law Rev* 2000;24: 541–568.

92. Wagatsuma H, Rosett A. The implications of apology: law and culture in Japan and the United States. *Law Soc Rev* 1986;20:461–496.

93. Robbennolt JK. Apologies and legal settlement: an empirical examination. *Mich Law Rev* 2003;102:460–516.

94. Rabin R. Dissembling and disclosing physician responsibility on the frontiers of tort law. *De Paul Law Rev* 2008;57:281–293.

95. Lazare A. The healing forces of apology in medical practice and beyond. *DePaul Law Rev* 2008;57:251–265.

96. Meadows KK. Resolving medical malpractice disputes in Massachusetts: statutory and judicial initiatives in alternative dispute resolution. *Suffolk J Trial Appellate Advocacy* 1999;4:165.

97. Jones J. Give a little whistle: the need for a more broad interpretation of the whistleblower exception to the employment-at-will doctrine. *Tex Tech Law Rev* 2003;34: 1133–1164.

98. Purtilo R. *Ethical Dimensions in the Health Care Professions*, 3rd ed. Philadelphia: W. B. Saunders; 1999.

99. Corbo J. *Kraus v. New Rochelle Hosp. Med. Ctr.*: Are whistleblowers finally getting the protection they need? *Hofstra Labor Employ Law J* 1994;12:141–162.

100. Bok S. Blowing the whistle. In: Fleishman J, Liebman L, Moore M, eds. *Public Duties: The Moral Obligation of Government Officials*. Cambridge, MA: Harvard Press; 1981, pp. 204–220.

101. *Peterman v. International Brotherhood of Teamsters (1963)*, 29 Cal. Rptr. 399.

102. Clark AD. Ethical implications of whistleblowing. *La Bus J* 1994;42:364.

103. Sarbanes-Oxley Act, *18 U.S.C. § 1514A*.

104. Ravishankar L. Encouraging Internal Whistleblowing in Organizations. Available at: http://www.scu.edu/ethics/publications/submitted/whistleblowing.html. Accessed March 31, 2009.

Safe Patient Care Systems

Kevin T. Fuji, Pat Hoidal, Kimberly A. Galt,
Andjela Drincic, and Amy A. Abbott

PURPOSE

The characteristics and practices of safe patient care systems are described in this chapter. How safety relates to the concepts of continuous quality improvement and total quality management is presented. Understanding the use of these tools to reduce patient harm and injury is a competency that all health professionals should have. The principles of patient safety place an emphasis on learning from actual errors and near misses to improve patient care systems. The role of patients and their caregivers as primary contributors to improving safe patient care systems is discussed.

OBJECTIVES

After completing this chapter, you will be able to:

- Describe the characteristics of a safe patient care system
- Discuss the concepts of total quality management and continuous quality improvement in the context of safe patient care systems
- Describe how healthcare teams learn from actual errors and near misses to promote a safe healthcare system
- Describe how patients can contribute to a safe patient care system

VIGNETTE

A middle-aged female was admitted to the hospital to have her gall bladder removed. After surgery, the surgeon informed her family that she was doing well in the recovery room. He ordered morphine (1 mg/hr as needed for pain) and Percocet (5/325 mg).

A few hours later, in her hospital room, the patient requested an increase in pain medication. Her nurse telephoned the surgeon, and a verbal order was given to increase the dose of morphine to 2 mg/hr as needed. The nurse returned to the patient's room and gave the patient 20 mg of morphine intravenously. The nurse thought that the dose she had given the patient seemed "a little high" and went to consult with a pharmacist who confirmed that the dose was too high. The nurse immediately contacted her nursing supervisor. At that point, the patient was rushed to the intensive care unit because she had stopped breathing. The patient was given an antidote and recovered with no long-term effects.

The surgeon was contacted. He explained to the patient and her family what had happened. He told the patient that she was given a higher dose of morphine than he had prescribed for her pain. He went on to explain the nurse who had made the mistake was very sorry and that she was the person who had saved the patient's life. The patient was understanding and released from the hospital with no further complications. The nurse was fired soon after.

IMPROVEMENTS IN PATIENT SAFETY

Lessons learned from using a systems approach to achieve quality in industry have applications for enhancing the safety and quality of patient care. By looking at past quality-improvement efforts, two distinct theories emerge. One theory focuses on the belief that identifying, blaming, and punishing individuals who make errors are the best ways to achieve quality. This theory assumes that the individual's performance is substandard and must be corrected or eliminated. The second theory, known as continuous improvement, suggests that quality problems primarily come from faulty procedures and processes, not from a lack of skill or learning on the part of individuals. The assumptions in this theory recognize that healthcare safety and quality are dependent on complex systems. Healthcare professionals have been encouraged to focus on the continuous improvement theory.[1]

THE SCIENCE OF SAFE SYSTEMS

The scientific study of human error is relatively new and involves disciplines such as cognitive psychology, human factors engineering, work group and organizational sociology, and systems analysis. Health professionals are typically unfamiliar with these disciplines, although great improvements in safety have come from the application of principles and insights from these "safety sciences." Lessons have been learned about the study of human error and normal cognitive function from the aviation industry. Well-known aviation accidents such as the Columbia Shuttle disaster illustrate slips, mistakes, errors in communication, and machine- or environment-aided errors. These underlying mechanisms of error in aviation can be applied to medicine.[2] Through analysis of accidents and near misses in aviation, nuclear power, and other related areas, much has been learned about how complex systems can be made to function more safely.

Systems analysis is a high-level view of the way things work and focuses on the idea that safety resides in the system, not in individuals, protocols, or devices. Systems analysis of accidents such as Three Mile Island and Chernobyl reveals that a single cause is almost never to blame. It is far more likely that multiple failures occur in a complex, interactive, unpredictable, and causal chain. Some of these failures may have been present in the system for months or years. These "latent failures" are properties of the system that facilitate the creation of active errors and failures by humans. Latent failures may be present in processes of design, management, resource allocation, and other areas. Mental slips or lapses by human workers in conjunction with these latent failures will either cause an active error or illuminate a system process that needs improvement. Some systems appear to be inherently more accident prone than others. These systems are often so complicated that normal processes within them produce a chain of events leading to a harmful outcome. This "normal accident" theory proposes that some accidents are truly the product of the system and that any attempt to identify a specific cause or blame an individual is misguided and unnecessary.[3]

A SYSTEMS CONTEXT FOR SAFETY

The Institute of Medicine report *To Err Is Human: Building a Safer Health System* focused the attention of the public, policy makers, and other healthcare stakeholders on patient safety issues.[4]

For many years, risk assessment and management experts have suggested that analysis of errors should not be focused solely on the individuals involved; however, when healthcare errors occur, there is a rush to attribute responsibility and blame to an individual. This is often overly simplistic, and although it promises a quick fix by providing a target for blame, it does not provide the answer to why the incident happened.

System interdependency exists at the point of care in all healthcare facilities. Systems factors create a context in which the provider must function—a context that can be error provoking. In contrast to popular assumption, actions of care providers do not emanate solely from their physiognomy (ergonomics) or their factors. Those factors include characteristics of the care recipient and the means of providing care, such as medical devices that interact with each other and with the characteristics of the provider. Although human errors are inevitable, a reduction of errors can be achieved through improvement of equipment design and a better understanding of human attitudes and behaviors in the context of their use.[2] These interactive interdependencies define the nucleus of the care-providing system. This system is embedded in systems of factors gleaned from taxonomies of error discussed by Senders and Moray and by Rasmussen and Rouse.[5,6] When clustered into categories, these factors can be envisioned as concentric circles of systems.

Systems range from those most proximal to the care-providing system (ambient conditions and physical and social environments), through the organization, to the most distal subsystems (legal–regulatory–reimbursement and cultural factors). Disturbances in any subsystem can affect any other system factors within its circumference, including the nuclear care-providing system. The most distal social policy subsystem can make the most pervasive impact.

When the care provider is assumed to be the source of error, information is collected about that person, not system factors, and the search ends. This is deceptive because healthcare errors are committed because contextual system factors create error-provoking situations and not because people are malicious. Focusing on the care provider as the sole source of error without considering the context does not effectively identify patient safety issues and distorts any analysis of what happened.

When errors occur, the context of care system must be identified and solutions formed. This system is analogous to the script of a performance; the care provider is the actor who responds to cues from other actors, props, and the setting. Although actors vary in talent, the script essentially determines their performance—replace actors and the performance changes little. Identify care providers as the error and remove them, and the context continues provoking error. A systems approach would address factors in the script, not in the performer. Health care must expand the search for error-provoking factors beyond the individual to the system of the context of care.[7]

QUALITY AND PATIENT SAFETY

The quality of health care is based on safe care, a relationship discussed as early as the mid-1800s. Based on her experience in hospitals in a number of countries, Florence Nightingale noted that "even admitting to the full extent the great value of the hospital improvements of recent years, a vast deal of the suffering, and some at least of the mortality, in these establishments is avoidable." She also noted that even in high-quality facilities, compromises in patient safety still occurred. More recently, the relationship between quality and safety has been described by the National Patient Safety Foundation, which noted, "Patient safety is related to 'quality of care,' but the two concepts are not synonymous. Safety is an important subset of quality." Quality of care and patient safety continue to challenge modern healthcare systems.[8]

Patient safety as a critical component of quality has been described in a two-dimensional model illustrating the influence of the external environment on quality. The first dimension identifies forces in the external environment that can prompt healthcare systems to engage in quality improvement (e.g., regulatory/legislative activities, economic incentives). The second dimension reflects three domains of quality: safe care, practice that is consistent with current medical knowledge, and customization.[4]

When assessing or measuring quality, three characteristics have been widely discussed, each of which can be related to patient safety. Quality includes the following:

- *Structure*: The capacity to provide high-quality care. This can include incorporation of resources in the system to protect patient safety (e.g., professional licensure).
- *Process (or performance)*: Clinical and technical aspects of care processes. This may include aspects that contribute to or compromise patient safety (e.g., drug administration errors).
- *Outcomes*: Changes in a patient's health status attributable to care processes (e.g., a number of patient falls in a healthcare facility). Outcomes can also be affected by the structure of a system.

The relationship between healthcare quality and patient safety can also be illustrated in the description of three different quality problems:

- *Overuse*: Unnecessary care that may put patient safety at risk (e.g., antibiotics).
- *Underuse*: Too little use of effective and appropriate care that can decrease unnecessary complications (e.g., prenatal care).

- *Misuse*: Inferior care resulting from inadequate performance by systems or healthcare providers that results in unnecessary injuries, delayed care, or mortality.

Preventable harm from medical treatment compromises patient safety and may result in injury, especially in the case of misuse.

Both internal and external efforts are used to promote healthcare quality and patient safety. External efforts may be in the form of regulations that are enacted to protect the public from unsafe care; however, this is often insufficient to ensure improvement in patient safety. At another level, characteristics of quality, such as decreased waiting time for appointments, may improve through competition between providers.

The main approaches used to improve quality that can also affect patient safety include quality-assurance (e.g., the use of patient surveys about the care they received while in the hospital) and quality-improvement efforts. Quality-assurance efforts are not always entirely effective, as evidenced by compromised patient safety stories in the news and from reports by federal oversight agencies. In contrast, quality-improvement efforts focus on facilitating quality improvement in a blame-free environment. Efforts are underway in healthcare facilities to improve quality around processes such as medication safety. Both approaches could be further adapted to improve patient safety and decrease medical errors.[9]

TOTAL QUALITY MANAGEMENT

Total quality management (TQM) is a management philosophy created by Dr. W. Edwards Deming, which emphasizes a commitment to excellence throughout the organization. Dr. Deming developed 14 points (Table 9–1) that provide the foundation for the Deming management method.[10] These principles of quality management were originally applied to improve quality and performance in the manufacturing industry. They are now widely used to improve quality and customer satisfaction in a number of service industries, including health care.

Characteristics of TQM

The four core characteristics of TQM are customer/client focus, total organizational involvement, the use of quality tools and statistics for measurement, and the identification of key processes for improvement.

Table 9-1 Deming's Management Method

1. Create constancy of purpose for improvement of product and service.
2. Adopt the new philosophy.
3. Cease dependence on mass inspection.
4. End the practice of awarding business based on price tag.
5. Improve constantly and forever the system of production and service.
6. Institute training.
7. Institute leadership.
8. Drive out fear.
9. Break down barriers between staff areas.
10. Eliminate slogans, exhortations, and targets for the workforce.
11. Eliminate numerical quotas.
12. Remove barriers to pride of workmanship.
13. Institute a vigorous program of education and retraining.
14. Take action to accomplish the transformation.

Data are from Koch MW, Fairly TM. *Integrated Quality Management: The Key to Improving Nursing Care Quality.* St. Louis: Mosby; 1993.

Customer/Client Focus

An important theme of quality management is to address the needs of customers. There are internal and external customers of healthcare organizations. Internal customers include employees and departments within the organization (e.g., the laboratory, admitting office, environmental services). External customers of a healthcare organization include patients, managed care organizations, insurance companies, and regulatory agencies (e.g., the Joint Commission on Accreditation of Healthcare Organizations [JCAHO], public health departments). Under the principles of TQM, it is important for the clinical manager to know who the customers are in order to meet their needs. Some healthcare examples are providing flexible schedules for employees, adjusting routines for morning care to meet the needs of patients, extending clinic hours, and putting infant changing tables in restrooms. Putting the customer first requires creative and innovative methods to meet the ever-changing needs of both internal and external customers.

Total Organizational Involvement

The goal of quality management is to involve all employees and empower them with the responsibility to make a difference in the quality of service they provide. This means that all employees must have knowledge of the TQM philosophy as it relates to their job and the overall goals and mission of the organization.

Knowledge of the TQM process breaks down barriers between departments and eliminates the phrase, "That's not my job." This means that clinical care personnel might clean a bed for a new admission from the emergency room or a physician might transport a patient to the radiology department.

The Use of Quality Tools and Statistics for Measurement

The use of quality tools and statistics for measurement are key components to improving quality. Many tools, formats, and designs can be used to build knowledge, make decisions, and improve quality. Tools for data analysis and display can be used to identify areas for process and quality improvement and then to benchmark the progress of improvements. Deming applied this scientific approach to the concept of TQM to develop the model seen in Figure 9–1 that he called the

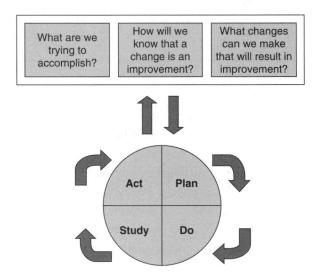

FIGURE 9–1 Model for Improvement

Data are from http://www.apiweb.org/services.htm#Developing_methods and http://www.ihi.org/IHI/Topics/Improvement/ImprovementMethods/HowToImprove; accessed March 2009. The Model for Improvement was developed by Associates in Process Improvement as a tool for accelerating improvement in systems. See Langley GL, Nolan KM, Nolan TW, Norman CL, Provost LP. *The Improvement Guide: A Practical Approach to Enhancing Organizational Performance*, 2nd ed. San Francisco: Jossey-Bass Publishers; 2009. The model has two parts: (1) three fundamental questions and (2) the Plan-Do-Study-Act (PDSA) cycle to test and implement changes in real work settings. The PDSA cycle guides the test of a change to determine if the change is an improvement. The PDSA cycle was originally developed by Walter A. Shewhart as the Plan-Do-Check-Act (PDCA) cycle. W. Edwards Deming modified Shewhart's cycle to PDSA, replacing "Check" with "Study."

PDCA cycle (Plan, Do, Check, and Act).[11] It is sometimes referred to as the Plan, Do, Study, Act cycle. In this cycle, a plan is created to carry out the processes needed to achieve a prespecified outcome (e.g., who, what, where, when, and how); the plan is implemented, and data are collected and analyzed. The actual outcomes are assessed against the prespecified outcomes, and changes that should be kept and changes that should be discarded are identified.

Identification of Key Processes for Improvement

All activities performed in an organization can be described in terms of processes. Processes within a healthcare setting can be systems related (e.g., admitting, discharging, and transferring patients), clinical (e.g., administering medications, managing pain), or clinical managerial (e.g., risk management and performance evaluations).[12] Complex processes involving multiple disciplines or departments should be examined closely to identify opportunities proactively to reduce inefficiencies, develop ways to improve performance, and promote positive outcomes.

CONTINUOUS QUALITY IMPROVEMENT

Within the philosophy of TQM, there is a methodology process, called continuous quality improvement (CQI), used to improve quality and performance. As the name implies, CQI is ongoing. It involves evaluations and actions that go beyond meeting standards and solving problems. This concept is sometimes challenging to relate to because patient care requires synchronizing activities across multiple departments; therefore, a well thought-out process is a key to a successful CQI are implementation.[13]

Role of CQI in Health Care

Continuous quality improvement moved health care from a mode of identifying failed standards, problems, and individuals to a proactive approach in which problems are prevented and ways to improve quality of care and patient safety are identified. This paradigm shift involves everyone in the delivery of patient care.

The Joint Commission and Performance Improvement Standards to Assure Safety

The Joint Commission identifies itself as an organization committed to patient safety. The commission identifies its own mission: to "continuously improve the safety and quality of care provided to the public through the provision of health care accreditation and related services that support performance improvement in health care organizations." The Joint Commission operates under the philosophy that accreditation is a risk-reduction activity and that compliance with standards is intended to reduce the risk of adverse outcomes. This is accomplished by assisting organizations by providing guidelines and standards that help focus quality-improvement efforts to both assure safety and promote improvements on an ongoing basis. The Joint Commission estimates that nearly 50% of its standards are focused on patient safety. Although these standards are broad based and subject to interpretation, their intent is to provide a framework for each healthcare organization to customize the process to meet its own circumstances and needs. The standards include specific requirements for the response to adverse events: the prevention of accidental harm through the analysis and redesign of vulnerable patient systems (e.g., the ordering, preparation, and dispensing of medications) and the organization's responsibility to tell a patient about the outcomes of the care provided to the patient—whether good or bad. In 2003, the JCAHO (now called The Joint Commission) established the National Patient Safety Goals. Each year since then these goals have been updated based on national feedback about progress that accredited organizations made toward achieving these goals.[14]

THE JOINT COMMISSION, PATIENT SAFETY COALITIONS, AND SAFETY IMPROVEMENT

A number of issues that affect patient safety challenge us to reach a common understanding of systems and problems in order to implement improvements. These challenges include sharing a common taxonomy for problem identification and communication, establishing innovative standardized protocols for patient safety solutions across organizations, measuring change as a result of incorporation of safety solutions, and involving patients and others who have experienced harm and injury or increased risk. Coalitions that are engaged in these different areas of safety improvement include the World Health Organization's World Alliance for Patient Safety (launched in October 2004), the National Coordinating Council on Medication Error Reporting & Prevention, the National Patient Safety Foundation, the National Quality Forum, Consumers Advancing Patient Safety, and "Champions for Patient Safety" a collaborative initiative of the leading United States patient safety organizations to begin harmonizing the numerous approaches to issues in patient safety.

COMPONENTS OF A COMPREHENSIVE QUALITY MANAGEMENT PROGRAM

The following steps are required to implement a quality management process to improve safety in a healthcare setting:

1. *Develop a comprehensive quality management plan.* A quality management plan is a systematic method to design, measure, assess, and improve organizational performance. It uses a multidisciplinary approach to identify processes and systems representing the goals and mission of the organization, customers, and opportunities for improvement.

2. *Set standards and benchmark.* Standards are statements that define a level of performance or set of conditions deemed acceptable by some authority. Standards relate to three major dimensions of quality care: structure, process, or outcome.[15]

   a. Structure standards relate to the physical environment, organization, and management of an organization.

   b. Process standards are those connected with the actual delivery of care.

   c. Outcome standards address the end result of care that has been given.

   An indicator is a tool used to measure the performance of structure, process, and outcome standards. It is objective and based on current knowledge. After indicators are identified, benchmarking, or comparing data with other internal and external reliable sources, is the key to quality improvement. In clinical care, standards are available from professional and specialty organizations; however, each organization and each patient care area must designate standards specific to the patient population being served. These standards are the foundation on which all other measures of quality are based.

   A clinical process standard might be this: "Immediately prior to administration of a medication to the patient, the nurse will perform a final check of the medication against the patient's name and medication orders to ensure that the correct medication is being administered to the correct patient at the correct time."

3. *Conduct performance appraisals.* Employee performance is evaluated based on requirements of the job. This feedback is essential for employees to be professionally accountable.

4. *Focus on interdisciplinary assessment and improvement.* There is always a need for groups to assess, analyze, and improve their own performance. Performance assessment methods should focus on the CQI philosophy, which involves group or interdisciplinary performance. Peer review is an example of interdisciplinary assessment (discussed later in the chapter).

CQI—HOW IT WORKS:
A PRACTICAL EXAMPLE

The following example describes how one hospital used quality-assessment activities to provide feedback information into the CQI process, with a goal of reducing length of stay for breast surgeries. A team consisting of physicians, surgeons, and clinicians was formed to examine the feasibility of this goal. The idea initially met much resistance. Surgeons were concerned about the potential for postoperative infection. Clinicians were concerned about the effective management of pain, and there was an overall concern about continuity of care; however, an investigation of infection rates revealed that no infections had occurred for the past 5 years. The team also determined that pain could be effectively managed with oral medications administered by the patient. Operating room clinicians were then consulted to determine whether a preoperative visit and postoperative follow-up system could be implemented. A system was implemented so that the same clinician would see the patient before surgery and for postoperative follow-up care. During the follow-up visit, the clinician also would give the patient a satisfaction survey to identify ways to improve the process from a patient's perspective.[16]

This example shows how CQI can work across disciplines and departments to improve the process in a specific area of health care. It also illustrates how data are collected within the hospital to guide the decision-making process (e.g., number of postoperative infections). Throughout the evaluation and implementation process, focus was on the patient. Implementation was continually evaluated using a patient satisfaction survey, which is one method used to monitor clinical care. Other common methods used include the clinical care audit, peer review, and utilization review.

Clinical audits can be retrospective or concurrent. A retrospective audit is conducted after a patient's discharge and involves examining large numbers of case records. The patient's entire course of care is evaluated, and comparisons are made across cases. Recommendations for change may be based on the experiences of many patients with similar care problems or also across the spectrum of care provided. In contrast, a concurrent audit is conducted during the patient's course of care. It examines and evaluates the care provided to achieve a desired therapeutic outcome, with the ability to make changes immediately based on the patient's evolving health status.

Peer review is a process that healthcare organizations use in order to assure that its healthcare professionals possess training and demonstrate competency to ensure the provision of safe and quality patient care. This objective process allows the organization to address deficiencies that may be present in education, skills, or policies and procedures that allow a healthcare professional to provide and manage safe, high-quality care effectively.

CQI AND A MAJOR ADVERSE EVENT

Major adverse events are one of the extreme indicators in a CQI program that trigger investigation procedures beyond collection of benchmark data. When a major event occurs, tools designed to focus on finding what is not working well in a process specifically related to the event itself are employed. The common tool used to discover process problems of this magnitude is Root Cause Analysis (RCA).

RCA is a quality-improvement tool originally designed by the U.S. Department of Energy to help organizations respond to an error and become proactive in prevention of future errors.[17] Root cause analysis was first established as a tool for analyzing inpatient errors. More recently, RCA has been used for analysis of sentinel events in outpatient settings.[18] It has been adopted in Veteran Administration systems since the mid-1990s, and to date, more than 7000 RCAs have been performed.[19] In addition, in 1997, the Joint Commission mandated the use of RCA in the investigation of sentinel events in accredited hospitals.[20] The Joint Commission is a strong proponent of using an RCA to improve quality of care and patient safety.

A root cause is a finding related to a process or system that reduces risk through a redesign. With foundations in industrial psychology and human factors engineering, it is a retrospective qualitative tool used for error analysis. Each root cause identified during an RCA should be addressed appropriately in order to improve the overall organization. An RCA is used to identify critical underlying reasons (root causes) leading to sentinel events, near misses, or events that repeatedly result in an error. A sentinel event is defined as an "unexpected occurrence involving death or serious physical or psychological injury or the risk thereof."[21] RCA not only explores active errors (those occurring at the point of human interface with the complex system) but furthers our understanding of latent errors, those representing failures of system design.[22,23]

An RCA is performed by first identifying the error or patient safety risk that needs to be addressed. An RCA should include following these steps:

1. Determine whether the incident warrants an RCA, keeping in mind the broader definition of a sentinel event described above.

2. Form an RCA team with a team leader. Individuals directly involved in the incident likely cannot be objective and should be excluded from the formal RCA team.

3. Collect the data. This step answers the question "what happened?" Data are collected through interviews, chart reviews, and document review. This results in a rich description of the event and determination of an accurate sequence of events and underlying conditions.

4. Analyze the data. This step answers the question "why did the error happen?" It focuses on both active and latent failures in different categories of factors that influence clinical practice such as institutional/regulatory, organizational/management, work environment, team factors, staff factors, task factors, and patient characteristics. Category labels may vary depending on the setting. It is frequently suggested to ask the question "why?" five times for each contributing cause. The analysis is frequently organized in the form of a tree ("Ishikawa") or fishbone diagram of factors leading to the event being analyzed.

5. Develop an action plan. The purpose of this step is to answer the third crucial question in error analysis: "What can we to do to prevent an error from happening again?" Specific recommendations for improvements need to be presented in addition to identifying administrative and systems changes that need to be undertaken.

6. Review outcome measures. These are necessary to evaluate the effectiveness of the RCA process and should be clear and quantifiable.

One of the more challenging steps in an RCA is to complete the data analysis. The question "why?" is asked (typically at least five times due to the complexity of healthcare systems) until no additional root causes can be identified. For example, if an RCA was conducted because a patient was administered an incorrect medication, the results might look like the following:

1. "Why?": The nurse did not double check the medication before administration.
2. "Why?": The nurse did not have enough time.
3. "Why?": A physician required the nurse's immediate help on another matter.
4. "Why?": There were no other nurses around on the floor.
5. "Why?": There is not enough nursing staff in the hospital.

This RCA revealed a number of different system areas or processes that could be improved across departments within the organization. Expertise from healthcare professionals belonging to a wide range of disciplines is necessary in order to address patient safety concerns that may be identified anywhere in an organization. The importance of a multidisciplinary perspective is apparent when examining the previous example. Although a nurse was centrally involved (and perhaps additional education needs to be provided to nursing staff to reinforce the importance of double-checking medications before administration), other disciplines also played a role in the error. Additional questions could also be asked about how the incorrect medication got into the nurse's hands in the first place (pharmacist) or why the nurse needed to divert her attention from the task at hand (physician). The JCAHO forms for investigating RCAs are provided in the Appendix at the end of this chapter.[24]

The use and effectiveness of RCA has been questioned.[25] When it comes to causing a shift in culture from individual blame to identifying system flaws, an RCA is likely fairly effective[19]; however, questions remain about an RCA's efficacy in error reduction. There are no studies in the peer-reviewed literature on effectiveness of RCA on patient safety. One of the most significant studies analyzed the efficacy of RCA in prevention of serious adverse drug events (ADEs) in a tertiary-care hospital in Texas over a 2-year period with an initial implementation period of 12 months and a 17-month follow-up phase.[26] In this institution, RCA analysis resulted in policy changes related to safety issues, including medication ordering and distribution processes as well as staffing levels. Results showed a 45% decrease in the rate of voluntarily reported serious ADEs between the study and follow-up periods. Although the authors attributed the decline in serious ADEs to the implementation of blame-free RCA, other factors may have contributed to the measured effect. From a methodologic standpoint, RCAs are uncontrolled case studies where bias (especially one caused by hindsight) could lead to inaccuracy in interpretation. There is no standardized RCA reporting resulting in variable quality of analysis itself.

Even in cases when an RCA is good at clarifying reasons behind an error, recommendations need to be of high quality and implementable, and outcomes need to be measurable in order to prevent future errors. Perhaps the weakest points of RCA are the last two steps of the process, developing an action plan and measuring outcomes.

Two common RCA recommendations in health care include re-education and writing a policy.[27] Those actions are not likely to result in significant error reduction. For example, events resulting from poorly constructed medical devices will be best prevented by redesign of the device rather than education efforts aimed at end-users.[18] Those solutions are hard to implement because of a lack of collaboration between stakeholders, including manufacturers and healthcare systems, but researchers are making attempts to raise awareness of this issue.[25]

In addition, unrealistic attempts to create absolute safety leading to overtly complex procedures that in themselves can lead to systems failures may be harmful. Finally, conducting an RCA is a time-consuming process that requires adequately trained personnel. It is estimated that each RCA requires 20 to 90 person hours to complete[25]; therefore, the lack of resources and time continue to be significant barriers, resulting in RCAs of poor quality.[28,29]

The purpose of RCAs is to examine systematically both active and latent errors, focusing on system failures causing adverse events or near misses. Although there are several limitations to an RCA, a well-done RCA may lead to improved patient safety by facilitating changes in healthcare systems. RCAs have serious limitations similar to other retrospective qualitative analysis methods.[30,31] When used in addition to other techniques employed in error reduction, an RCA remains an important tool to help us learn from past mistakes.

PATIENT INVOLVEMENT IN QUALITY IMPROVEMENT

Patients have inherited more responsibility for safety in healthcare delivery today. As the consumer of health care, the patient is the primary source of information about how safe care is and what the quality of care is. Direct involvement in the quality improvement process has become a mainstay in health care. In order for healthcare professionals to understand patient needs, patients must communicate deficiencies, or negative experiences, they have or observe during their course of care.

Patients may also be involved in many of the organizational activities that have been identified through the CQI philosophy and the TQM process. For example, patient satisfaction surveys can be an important component of a quality-improvement program. Such a survey solicits patient perceptions on quality of care received and may provide suggestions for improvements.

A source of information to promote direct participation by patients in safe care includes the Agency for Healthcare Research and Quality website.[32] Some of the patient safety tools provided on this site include patient and caregiver guides to help get better quality care, patient versions of clinical practice guidelines to help the patient better understand the quality of care being provided compared to published standards, and how to prevent medication errors.

Another source of information is the major consumer advocacy and education group Consumers Advancing Patient Safety, a national consumer-led organization formed to be a collective voice for individuals, families, and healers who suffer harm in healthcare encounters. This organization offers much education and information to consumers who want to engage directly in advancing safety improvements.[33]

Despite the attention on improving patient safety, the patient frequently remains invisible to healthcare professionals during an episode of care. An ongoing theme expressed by patients is that healthcare professionals do not listen to them or to their concerns.[34] Healthcare professionals could enhance their relationship with patients by actively engaging patients during an episode of care. This may involve ensuring that patients and their caregivers understand the treatment being provided and have an opportunity to voice any questions or concerns they may have.

Patients have been encouraged to be responsible for their health care but are vulnerable when they are sick. Vulnerability can range from physical difficulty with communication to cultural differences in how illness is managed. This vulnerability is an important characteristic for healthcare professionals to be aware of and respect. Having the patient bring along an advocate has been proposed as a way to address the vulnerability of a sick patient. The patient advocate can ask questions to help to ensure that patient needs are being met. Organizations such as the Agency for Healthcare Research and Quality and Consumers Advancing Patient Safety provide resources so that patients, caregivers, and advocates can be prepared to understand what should happen during an episode of care and ways to communicate with healthcare professionals if questions or concerns arise.

SUMMARY

Quality management is the method by which performance of care is evaluated and improved. The principles of TQM include a focus on the customer (patient), empowerment of employees, and the collective work of the team. The philosophy of TQM can be carried out through a CQI program, which is a prevention-focused approach that provides the basis for managing risk. Improvement is established in a CQI through the use of standards that define an acceptable level of performance and benchmarking to track the progress of improvements. Tools such as clinical audits, outcomes management, and RCA are used to identify system processes for improvement, provide solutions for problems that are identified, and produce continual feedback on improvements that have been implemented.

A CLOSING CASE

Marie Wilson is a middle-aged, white woman with a 26-year history of type 1 diabetes mellitus.[18] She had used an insulin pump for 14 years; however, her diabetes was suboptimally controlled, and the decision was made to upgrade her insulin pump. When Marie received the new pump, she contacted the clinic to set up an appointment to meet with the nurse practitioner, who was a certified diabetes educator and pump trainer. Because Marie was eager to start using the new pump, the training appointment was added to an already full clinic day. The clinic had no formal policies and procedures for initiating or upgrading insulin pump therapy. The patient programmed the pump with direct nurse practitioner supervision. The patient manually primed the new pump according to the procedure she used to prime her old pump, and, with a blood sugar of more than 300 mg/dL, acted to deliver a bolus of rapid-acting insulin via the new pump. The patient then left the clinic to go to a meeting, but agreed to return later that day to meet with the nurse practitioner and the pump company representative (Representative A). The patient's blood sugar was 467 mg/dL when she returned to the clinic that afternoon, and she administered a bolus of rapid-acting insulin subcutaneously by syringe. The nurse practitioner questioned a potential delivery problem and contacted the pump company's help desk, who verified the settings and informed the nurse practitioner that a blood sugar of 300 would take awhile to come down. The patient left the clinic stating that she felt comfortable with the new pump. Representative A arrived at the clinic after the patient had left and reviewed questions with the nurse practitioner. The nurse practitioner asked Representative A to follow up with the patient that evening to check on her high blood sugars and to answer questions about the new pump. He arranged for another company representative (Representative B) to do so. When Representative B contacted the patient that evening, the patient's blood sugar had come down to around 200 mg/dL. The patient told Representative B that she felt like she was doing well with the pump. At bedtime, the patient's blood sugar was >250 mg/dL, at which point she gave herself another bolus of insulin via the pump. The following morning, the patient contacted the physician to report severe nausea, vomiting, and a high blood sugar. The physician sent her to the emergency department, where she was admitted and treated for diabetic ketoacidosis. Representative B was asked to go to the hospital and evaluate the pump. She determined that the pump had been improperly primed, resulting in no insulin delivery.

1. What would be an appropriate quality-improvement tool to address this incident?

2. What are the root causes leading to patient safety problems in this case?
3. What are some system improvements that could be implemented to address the identified root causes?

Discussion Questions to Launch Further Investigation

For further investigation, seek answers to these questions:

1. Describe how continuous quality improvement differs from quality assurance.
2. What is the clinician's role in addressing the various *types* of healthcare risks?
3. What is the patient's role in the quality improvement process?

REFERENCES

1. Berwick DM. Continuous improvement as an ideal in health care. *N Engl J Med* 1989;320:53–56.
2. Allnutt MF. Human factors in accidents. *Br J Anaesth* 1987;59:856–864.
3. Wears RL. The science of safety. In: Zipperer LA, Cushman S, eds. *Lessons in Patient Safety*. Chicago: National Patient Safety Foundation; 2001.
4. Kohn LT, Corrigan JM, Donaldson MS, eds. *To Err Is Human: Building a Safer Health System*. Washington, DC: National Academy Press; 2000.
5. Senders J, Moray N. *Human Error: Cause, Prediction, and Reduction*. Hillsdale, NJ: Lawrence Erlbaum Associates; 1991.
6. Rasmussen J, Rouse WB, eds. *Human Detection and Diagnosis of System Failures*. New York: Plenum Press; 1980.
7. Bogner MS, Roberts KH. A systems context for safety. In: Zipperer LA, Cushman S, eds. *Lessons in Patient Safety*. Chicago: National Patient Safety Foundation; 2001.
8. The National Patient Safety Foundation. National Agenda for Action: Patients and Families in Patient Safety. Available at: http://www.npsf.org/download/AgendaFamilies.pdf. Accessed March 27, 2009.
9. Wakefield MK. The relationship between quality and patient safety. In: Zipperer LA, Cushman S, eds. *Lessons in Patient Safety*. Chicago: National Patient Safety Foundation; 2001.
10. Koch MW, Fairly TM. *Integrated Quality Management: The Key to Improving Nursing Care Quality*. St. Louis: Mosby; 1993.
11. Institute for Healthcare Improvement. Improvement Methods. Available at: http://www.ihi.org/IHI/Topics/Improvement/ImprovementMethods/HowToImprove. Accessed March 24, 2009.
12. Schroeder PS. *Improving Quality and Performance: Concepts, Programs, and Techniques*. St. Louis: Mosby; 1994.
13. Migrant Clinicians Network. Quality Management Plan. Available at: http://www.migrantclinician.org/files/resourcebox/CQIPlan5.pdf. Accessed March 24, 2009.
14. The Joint Commission. Facts About Patient Safety. Available at: http://www.jointcommission.org/PatientSafety/facts_patient_safety.htm. Accessed March 24, 2009.

15. Bernstein SJ, Hilborne LH. Clinical indicators: the road to quality care? *Jt Comm J Qual Improv* 1993;19(11):501–509.

16. Wakefield DS, Wakefield BJ. Overcoming the barriers to implementation of TQM/CQI in hospitals: myths and realities. *QRB Qual Rev Bull* 1993;19(3):83–88.

17. U.S. Department of Energy. Root Cause Analysis Guidance Document. Available at: http://www.hss.doe.gov/nuclearsafety/ns/techstds/standard/nst1004/nst1004.pdf. Accessed March 25, 2009.

18. Rule AM, Drincic A, Galt KA. New technology, new errors: how to prime an upgrade of an insulin infusion pump. *Jt Comm J Qual Patient Saf* 2007;33(3):155–162.

19. Bagian JP, Gosbee J, Lee CZ, Williams L, McKnight SD, Mannos DM. The Veterans Affairs root cause analysis system in action. *Jt Comm J Qual Improv* 2002;28(10): 531–545.

20. The Joint Commission. Sentinel Event Policy and Procedures. Available at: http://www.jointcommission.org/SentinelEvents/PolicyandProcedures/se_pp.htm. Accessed March 31, 2009.

21. The Joint Commission. Sentinel Event. Available at: http://www.jointcommission.org/ SentinelEvents/. Accessed March 31, 2009.

22. Reason J. *Human Error.* New York: Cambridge University Press, 1990.

23. Reason J. Human error: models and management. *BMJ* 2000;320:768–770.

24. The Joint Commission. Sentinel event forms and tools. Available at: http://www. jointcommission.org/SentinelEvents/Forms. Accessed March 25, 2009.

25. Wu AW, Lipshutz AKM, Peter J, Pronovost PJ. Effectiveness and efficiency of root cause analysis in medicine. *JAMA* 2008;299:685–687.

26. Rex JH, Turnbull JE, Allen SJ, Vande Voorde K, Luther K. Systematic root cause analysis of adverse drug events in a tertiary referral hospital. *Jt Comm J Qual Improv* 2000;26:563–575.

27. Mills PD, Neily J, Luan D, Osborne A, Howard K. Actions and implementation strategies to reduce suicidal events in the Veterans Health Administration. *Jt Comm J Qual Patient Saf* 2006;32(3):130–141.

28. Braithwaite J, Westbrook MT, Mallock NA, Travaglia JF, Iedema RA. Experiences of health professionals who conducted root cause analyses after undergoing a safety improvement program. *Qual Saf Health Care* 2006;15:393–399.

29. Wallace LM, Spurgeon P, Earll L. *Evaluation of the NPSA's 3 Day RCA Programme: Report to the Department of Health Patient Safety Research Programme.* Coventry, England: Coventry University; 2006.

30. Giacomini MK, Cook DJ. Users' guides to the medical literature: XXIII. Qualitative research in health care A. Are the results of the study valid? Evidence-Based Medicine Working Group. *JAMA* 2000;284:357–362.

31. Giacomini MK, Cook DJ. Users' guides to the medical literature: XXIII. Qualitative research in health care B. What are the results and how do they help me care for my patients? Evidence-Based Medicine Working Group. *JAMA* 2000;284:478–482.

32. Agency for Healthcare Research and Quality. Consumers and patients. Available at: http://www.ahrq.gov/consumer. Accessed March 25, 2009.

33. Consumers Advancing Patient Safety. Available at: http://www.patientsafety.org. Accessed March 25, 2009.

34. Chassin MR, Becher EC. The wrong patient. *Ann Intern Med* 2002;136:826–833.

Appendix
Root Cause Analysis Tool

Level of Analysis		Questions	Findings	Root Cause?	Ask "Why?"	Take Action?
What happened?	Sentinel Event	What are the details of the event (brief description)?				
		When did the event occur (date, day of week, time)?				
		What area/service was impacted?				
Why did it happen?	The process or activity in which the event occurred.	What are the steps in the process, as designed (a flow dia-gram may be helpful here)?				
What were the most proximate factors?		What steps were involved in (contributed to) the event?				
(Typically "special cause" variation)	Human factors	What human factors were relevant to the outcome?				
	Equipment factors	How did the equipment performance affect the outcome?				
	Controllable environmental factors	What factors directly affected the outcome?				

APPENDIX 183

	Uncontrollable external factors	Are they truly beyond the organization's control?				
	Other	Are there any other factors that have directly influenced this outcome?				
		What other areas or services are impacted?				

This template is provided as an aid in organizing the steps in a root cause analysis. Not all possibilities and questions will apply in every case, and there may be others that will emerge in the course of the analysis; however, all possibilities and questions should be fully considered in your quest for "root cause" and risk reduction.

As an aid to avoiding "loose ends," the three columns on the right are provided to be checked off for later reference:

- "Root Cause?" should be answered "yes" or "no" for each finding. A root cause is typically a finding related to a process or system that has a potential for redesign to reduce risk. If a particular finding that is relevant to the event is not a root cause, be sure that it is addressed later in the analysis with a "why?" question. Each finding that is identified as a root cause should be considered for an action and addressed in the action plan.
- "Ask 'Why?'" should be checked off whenever it is reasonable to ask why the particular finding occurred (or didn't occur when it should have)—in other words, to drill down further. Each item checked in this column should be addressed later in the analysis with a "why?" question. It is expected that any significant findings that are not identified as root causes themselves have "roots."
- "Take Action?" should be checked for any finding that can reasonably be considered for a risk reduction strategy. Each item checked in this column should be addressed later in the action plan. It will be helpful to write the number of the associated Action Item on page 3 in the "Take Action?" column for each of the findings that requires an action.

Level of Analysis	Questions	Findings	Root Cause?	Ask "Why?"	Take Action?
Human Resources issues	To what degree are staff members properly qualified and currently competent for their responsibilities?				
Why did that happen? What systems and processes underlie those proximate factors?	How did actual staffing compare with ideal levels?				
(Common cause variation here may lead to special cause variation in dependent processes)	What are the plans for dealing with contingencies that would tend to reduce effective staffing levels?				
	To what degree is staff performance in the operant process(s) addressed?				
	How can orientation and in-service training be improved?				

184

Category	Question							
Information management issues	To what degree is all necessary information available when needed? Accurate? Complete? Unambiguous?							
	To what degree is communication among participants adequate?							
Environmental management issues	To what degree was the physical environment appropriate for the processes being carried out?							
	What systems are in place to identify environmental risks?							
	What emergency and failure-mode responses have been planned and tested?							
Leadership issues: Corporate culture	To what degree is the culture conducive to risk identification and reduction?							
Encouragement of communication	What are the barriers to communication of potential risk factors?							
Clear communication of priorities	To what degree is the prevention of adverse outcomes communicated as a high priority? How?							
Uncontrollable factors	What can be done to protect against the effects of these uncontrollable factors?							

Action Plan	Risk-Reduction Strategies	Measures of Effectiveness
For each of the findings identified in the analysis as needing an action, indicate the planned action expected, implementation date, and associated measure of effectiveness OR	Action Item 1:	
If after consideration of such a finding, a decision is made not to implement an associated risk reduction strategy, indicate the rationale for not taking action at this time.	Action Item 2:	
Check to be sure that the selected measure will provide data that will permit assessment of the effectiveness of the action.	Action Item 3:	
Consider whether pilot testing of a planned improvement should be conducted.	Action Item 4:	
Improvements to reduce risk should ultimately be implemented in all areas where applicable, not just where the event occurred. Identify where the improvements will be implemented.	Action Item 5:	
	Action Item 6:	
	Action Item 7:	
	Action Item 8:	
Cite any books or journal articles that were considered in developing this analysis and action plan:		

CHAPTER 10

The Use of Evidence to Improve Safety

Kimberly A. Galt and John M. Gleason

PURPOSE

This chapter examines the concept of evidence as it is applied to patient safety. The need to expand the definition of evidence to include qualitative, quantitative, and mixed-methods approaches to gathering evidence and accepting the validity and usefulness of these findings is examined. Implications to patient safety resultant from recognition and consideration of different evidence-based approaches are explored.

OBJECTIVES

After completing this chapter, you will be able to:

- Discuss the concept of evidence as applied to patient safety
- Describe the different knowledge forms of evidence that we use in patient safety
- Discuss reliability, validity, and levels of evidence as applied to patient safety
- Describe how to use different forms of evidence appropriately for the right questions in patient safety
- Describe the outcomes that may potentially occur when evidence is used inappropriately in safety decisions
- Become familiar with federal patient safety organizations

VIGNETTE

Lucía works as a certified nursing assistant (CNA) at a long-term care facility. When she arrives for each shift, she is assigned a number from one to six. For each number, there is a list of assigned residents and important things to remember about each resident (e.g., whether the resident has dentures or hearing aids, the type of incontinence product used, whether an alarm is used with the resident, and the location where meals are eaten).

One night when Lucía was working, the CNAs on the shift had completed their tasks for the night and were charting. The charge nurse did her final medication pass and checked that the CNAs had completed their responsibilities with each resident. The nurse observed nothing unusual and returned to the nurse's station to finish her charting.

When the next shift of CNAs began work, they did their first rounds to make sure all of the residents were clean and safe. As one CNA entered a room, she found the resident, Marie, lying on the ground. Marie was not able to walk but always insisted that she could. Because she was at risk for falling, she was required to wear an alarm that would sound when she tried to stand from her chair or bed. On this night, the CNA had not placed the alarm on Marie's arm, and the nurse missed this during her final rounds. Fortunately, Marie sustained only minor bruises and had no long-term effects from the fall.

Lucía was upset the next day when she learned that Marie had fallen. She felt badly that she had made a mistake. She talked to the charge nurse who also felt badly that she had missed the fact that Marie's alarm had not been set. Together, they went to the director of nursing to suggest that a root cause analysis be done to see whether this could be prevented in the future. The director of nursing said that there was no evidence to suggest that a root cause analysis was effective in improving patient safety and that they did not have enough staff time to conduct one. She told Lucía and the charge nurse to be more careful.

WHAT CONSTITUTES EVIDENCE IN SAFETY?

A substantive debate about what constitutes evidence in patient safety has been occurring for well over a decade.[1,2] It was over 10 years ago that the finding of over a million injuries secondary to medical mistakes occurred in the United States annually, with 100,000 deaths as a result. A public outcry resulted, and the government, professionals, healthcare organizations, and consumers rallied to find solutions to make health care safer.

Historically, evidence-based approaches have been regarded as the most appropriate way to make medical care decisions for patients. If true, then what is central to this debate? The essence of the debate is this: Which form or forms of evidence are acceptable, and how much of this evidence is enough to say, "Good enough; let's make this change"?

When we design inquiries to respond to our questions with a high level of rigor, this gives us the confidence that we need to make system changes. The traditional rigor comes from grounding our studies in statistically sound frameworks. This includes studies that can be described through the use of random sampling procedures and adequate sample sizes to achieve answering the research question at the 95% confidence level (we will only draw a different conclusion 1 of 20 times that we conduct the study). It has been particularly difficult to make sound decisions on the local level and in daily work in health care about improvements to systems to adopt in patient safety because there is a minimal body of evidence that has the traditional rigor we usually seek from scientific studies to inform us about patient safety problems and solutions.

We therefore benefit by understanding evidence from various points of view and its various forms and uses. We need to work with the forms of evidence accessible to us and to learn to structure inquiry to inform us in the context of our needs for patient safety. Not all patient safety questions need to be answered through rigorous randomized controlled trials. They do need to be answered in a contextually relevant way, using approaches that give us confidence in the findings so that we may use these findings to make safety improvement decisions in our work.

Sources of Evidence

Evidence may emerge from the published literature, as well as from data collected in a wide range of settings and interpreted for meaningful findings by stakeholders who are engaged in the processes of care; however, important information that we use in making decisions is also commonly found in the form of tacit knowledge and anecdote—generated for use by others and deemed "good enough" to use in decision making and practice improvement initiatives. This is the most common way we make decisions on a daily basis.

Knowledge Forms, Paradigms, and Perceptions

The importance of conducting contextually relevant research to gain needed knowledge for improving safety cannot be overstated; however, this knowledge exists in varying forms and among persons with their own way of understanding its meaning. Individual people perceive the "same" thing from a singular, individual point of view. This concept is amplified in patient safety because many of the safety problems emerge from complex systems, and some involve complex therapies and complex systems simultaneously. Although we publish and share knowledge for others to use, this knowledge is often positioned as a component that emerged from a single viewpoint among several persons' viewpoints of constituents who "own the knowledge," or we each have a point of view, or a lens, with which we see things that are relatively unique to oneself. In a sense, we each have our own set of paradigms or glasses through which we view the world. These personal viewpoints of the "way things are" may cloud our ability to perceive or consider new or different ideas, especially if they seem to be in conflict with our perception of what is reality or "truth." In 1962, Thomas Kuhn wrote *The Structure of Scientific Revolutions*, in which he developed the concept of a "paradigm shift." Kuhn argues that scientific advancement is not evolutionary, but rather is a "series of peaceful interludes punctuated by intellectually violent revolutions." In those revolutions, "one conceptual world view is replaced by another."[3] A paradigm shift may be thought of as a change from one way of thinking to another. It does not just happen, but rather, it is usually driven by agents of change. We believe that this idea is relevant with the paradigm shift that has occurred socially with the emergent priority of improving patient safety in health care.

This has implications for our ability to acknowledge what is acceptable evidence and the methodologic approaches we use to gather it and interpret it. To answer complex inquiries about safety, we are challenged to structure research designs that can capture knowledge, or evidence, in a meaningful way for each person who will use it and interpret it. This meaningfulness is translated at individual and local environment levels, group or organizational levels, and system levels. To accumulate meaningful knowledge, we need to explore the complex question often present in patient safety by breaking down central questions into subquestions; addressing questions grounded in multiple theories and disciplines; combining sequenced or embedded qualitative and quantitative approaches; and addressing multiple contexts that emerge through the viewpoints of individuals who will use this information. This suggests that many forms of knowledge should be acceptable as evidence to aid decisions to improve safety.

The traditional methods that we have used, although reliable and valid, are too narrow to satisfy the wide range of safety improvement needs that we have today. We are experiencing evidentiary "tensions" and "tugs." Most of us in patient safety research today recognize that we are not satisfied with our progress and how it is going.

How will we address this need? More and more agreement seems to be present that suggests that we need to use qualitative methods, quantitative methods, and most recently mixed methods to attain our evidence. The research method called "mixed methods" has great potential to assist us in meeting this challenge. Mixed methods approaches to inquiry provide the opportunity to employ the creativity in a research design that is required to address these complex questions. A design should provide a research process that best meets the purpose of the research. The mixed methods approach to the research process provides a cognitive structure to how we can combine, sequence, or embed qualitative and quantitative methods of data collection, analysis, and interpretation. Table 10–1 displays differing research designs and methods that are considered sound approaches to gathering evidence in the three design traditions.

Reliability of Evidence

We should always consider the extent of reliability of the evidence we are considering. Reliable evidence suggests that each time we make the same change to

Table 10–1 Contemporary Strategies of Inquiry Recognized by Various Disciplines that Could Be Applied to Gathering Evidence for Use in Patient Safety Improvement

Quantitative	Qualitative	Mixed Method
Experimental	Grounded Theory	Action Research
• Between-group designs	• Systematic	• Practical
• Within-group designs	• Emerging	• Participatory
Quasi-experimental	• Constructivist	• Community based
Correlation	Ethnographic	Mixed Designs
• Explanatory	• Realistic	• Triangulation
• Prediction	• Critical	• Embedded
Survey	• Case study	• Sequential
• Cross-sectional	Narrative research	○ Explanatory
• Longitudinal	Biography	○ Exploratory
Modeling	Phenomenology	
• Regression	Case Study	
• Hierarchical linear		
• Structural equation		

Courtesy of Kimberly A. Galt © 2008.

improve safety we will see the same result almost all of the time. For example, if we use error-reporting data, we may find that the limitations of present reporting systems and methods are likely to generate data that are not likely to be similar from one time period to the next. Similarly, the data reported from one system or hospital are systematically likely to be different in structure from another system or hospital. This takes us back to the "apples and oranges" problem discussed in Chapter 4. Another limitation that challenges reliability is the voluntary nature of error reporting. Even the national reporting system, the FDA MedWatch program, is a voluntary system; therefore, the frequency of events by type is not systematically examined nationally. We need to continue to improve our methods to overcome these limitations to gain the knowledge needed for some improvements. This is further evidenced by the recent literature focusing on the emerging methods being used for comparative effectiveness and safety questions.[4]

Validity of Evidence

Valid evidence represents what we actually think it represents. Is the evidence we are seeing, for example, a reported adverse drug event multiple times in multiple patients, characterized by the same traits? Are observers seeing an event and categorizing the events the same, when actually they are very different occurrences? We should therefore accept *types of evidence* appropriate for the question that we are asking. Qualitative evidence can be confirmatory (i.e., the story is sometimes all we need). Alternatively, quantitative evidence can be exploratory (i.e., measures and metrics may only identify the problem, not the solution, more clearly).

Appropriate Use of Evidence

Traditional means of looking at evidence suggests that testing a hypothesis using a randomized controlled trial is the strongest evidence one can accumulate to support an idea; however, these are expensive, lengthy, and difficult experiments to conduct. As a result, some questions that beg an answer using this level of rigor are impractical or sometimes impossible to answer. We must determine when we have enough evidence of a level of strength that is sufficient for making decisions to improve patient safety; therefore, we must accept *levels of evidence* that are "good enough." For example, descriptive findings can be powerful evidence for the right question. This form of evidence is used in root cause analysis studies to explore how to improve a system after a major error or accident has occurred (see Chapter 9).

Evaluation of the Strength of the Evidence

The Agency for Healthcare Research and Quality financially supported the development of the UCSF-Stanford Evidence-based Practice Center (EPC) evidence report. This report takes the approach of providing definitions of levels of evidence. Level 1, the strongest level, is randomized controlled trials. Level 2 is nonrandomized controlled trials. Level 3 is observational studies with controls, for example, cohort studies with controls and case-control studies. Level 4 is observational studies without controls, for example, cohort studies without controls and case series. Systematic reviews and meta-analyses were assigned to the highest level of study design included in the review. This hierarchy does not contain the usual lower levels of evidence included in most evidence hierarchies of multiple time series studies and expert opinion. The UCSF-Stanford EPC further defined an outcome measure hierarchy with level 1 as clinical outcomes (e.g., morbidity, mortality, adverse events), level 2 as surrogate outcomes, level 3 as other measurable variables with an indirect or unestablished connection to the target safety outcome, and level 4 as no outcomes relevant to decreasing medical errors and/or adverse events.[5] Although not all experts use this approach, it provides a framework for consideration as we continue to improve in our ability to determine the strength and usefulness of our research findings.

WHEN TO USE METHODS OF HIGH RIGOR

Some questions are of such importance to answer correctly that traditional models of rigor (e.g., the randomized controlled trial) are minimally required. For example, the answer to the high stakes question "how does the use of a hand-held personal digital assistant (PDA) for prescribing and accessing drug information at the point of care impact potential prescribing errors?" is important both humanistically and economically. In a study conducted by Creighton University researchers, the impact of hand-held devices on prescribing revealed outcomes related to prescription omissions, commissions, and legibility.[6,7]

This was the largest study to date to evaluate the impact of ambulatory computerized provider order entry (ACPOE). The study examined 78 practitioners in 31 primary care outpatient practices who were provided a basic, stand-alone ACPOE system using hand-held technology (PDAs) with drug information support and the ability to determine the presence of interactions between a patient's medications. None of the office sites had clinical computing in the patient examination rooms nor fully integrated office management systems, demanding that the ACPOE system stand alone from these systems.

This randomized controlled trial demonstrated that a substantial improvement in prescription legibility, prescription omissions, and reduction in abbreviation and symbol use (antecedents to errors) occurs with ACPOE using hand-held PDA devices. Table 10–2 displays the results of this study. Overall illegibility of the prescriptions decreased from 9.1% to 2.7%. All types of errors attributable to omission on the prescription were reduced. The omission of the patient's age or birth date dropped from 95.5% of prescriptions at baseline to 59.2% after PDA introduction.[6]

These findings were not possible to learn without using a randomized controlled trial design. To answer this question with less rigor would likely result in failure to learn meaningful results, an unfortunate impact on patients. The cost

Table 10–2 Impact of Partial Adoption of PDA Intervention on Prescription Errors

Percentage Error in Intervention Group (Baseline) (n = 19,372 Rx)	Percentage Error in Intervention Group (Post-PDA Use) (n = 14,378 Rx)*	Type of Error
76.6	17.7	Illegible prescriber signature
55.9	27.6	Unclear prescriber identity
18.7	9.8	Illegible patient name
9.1	2.7	Illegible prescription overall
0.6	0.1	Omission of patient name
95.5	59.2	Omission of patient age or birth date
99.8	99.7	Omission of patient address
1.4	0.6	Omission of date prescription written
1.3	1.3	Omission of prescriber signature[†]
89.9	78.5	Omission of indication for medication
18.5	12.1	Omission of prescription refill status
0.5	0.2	Omission of drug name
20.9	17.0	Omission of drug strength
84.7	51.7	Omission of dosage form
6.2	4.5	Omission of quantity to dispense or duration of treatment

(continues)

13.4	11.7	Omission of drug dose
30.8	19.5	Omission of route of administration
5.3	4.8	Omission of schedule for administration
3.4	2.3	Use of an abbreviation for the drug name
61	70.5	Use of an abbreviation for the dose amount‡
1.6	0.5	Use of an abbreviation for the quantity
63.2	36.7	Use of an abbreviation for the route of administration
85.8	50.7	Use of an abbreviation for frequency of administration
76.7	47.4	Use of symbols on face of prescription
0.4	0.3	Use of a trailing zero after a decimal point
0.5	0.4	No use of a leading zero before a decimal point
9.4	11.1	Vagueness of instructions on prescription
0	0.3	Wrong route of drug administration on prescription

*Forty-three percent of prescriptions were generated through the PDA.
†No electronic signature was used in this study.
‡E-prescribing application used abbreviations for some dose amounts.
From Galt KA, Rule A, Taylor W, et al. Impact of personal digital assistant devices on medication safety in primary care. *AHRQ Advances in Patient Safety: From Research to Implementation* [serial on CD-ROM]. Rockville, MD: Agency for Healthcare Research and Quality; 2005;3:247–263.

to convert a primary care office to support this technology if proven useful in a fully integrated manner is 0.75 to 1 million dollars for a small independent office. This is not a repeatable mistake for most practices.

This study, however, also illustrates that using qualitative interviews through direct observation in this field study of only one group, the PDA users, was a powerful approach to learning about the barriers and solutions to technology and did not require being a part of the randomized control trial. It did require the use of qualitative observation and analysis techniques on the right subjects. A direct observation study using interviews identified technology readiness of both the users and the primary care office systems as a major component to successful adoption.[6]

Table 10–3 displays these results. Areas of improvement identified through this research indicate the need to customize ACPOE to the office workflow and user needs, the lack of system integration with other computerized support systems, the lack of complete accommodation (i.e., less than 100% of medication prescriptions that can be generated via technology), users circumventing the system because it is so easy to write prescriptions by hand, standardization of computer technology operating system platforms between offices, accommodation of prescribing systems to gradual user adoption, and tracking of and new types of

---

Table 10–3 Physician-Reported Barriers and Solutions Themes

Barriers Themes	Solutions Themes
Technology	**Individual level**
• *Hardware*—The time it took for the prescription to print perceived to be increased.	• *Self-help*—Physician takes an active role in solving the problem and continues to try using the PDA.
• *Software*—The prescription-generation tool perceived to be cumbersome.	• *Partial adoption*—Physician incorporates and continues to use only the applications of the PDA that work best for his practice.
Time	
• *Learning time*—The time needed to learn how to use the PDA.	• *Avoidance*—Physician essentially gives up on using the PDA partly because the perceived workload does not allow her to seek a solution.
• *Prescription generation*—The time needed to write and print the prescription using the PDA.	
• *Workload*—The perceived patient volume of the physician that day.	**System level**
Environment	• *System redesign*—Physician proposes that the solution requires an organizational commitment and investment to improving the clinic environment to promote use of the PDA.
• *Technology ready*—Offices are not ready or equipped properly to support the prescribing and printing system.	
• *Printer location*—Printers were not conveniently located so as not to disrupt workflow.	• *Organizational development*—Physician proposes that the solution requires the organization to recognize the need for and support the necessary training and development.
Personal views	
• *Patient centeredness*—The use of the PDA or its software was not appropriate for the patient mix of the clinic.	
• *Slow to adapt*—Interest level or fear of technology slowed adoption.	

From Galt KA, Rule A, Taylor W, et al. Impact of personal digital assistant devices on medication safety in primary care. *AHRQ Advances in Patient Safety: From Research to Implementation* [serial on CD-ROM]. Rockville, MD: Agency for Healthcare Research and Quality; 2005;3:247–263.

errors secondary to technology. Despite these issues, basic systems of ACPOE (PDA with a drug information source) demonstrate value through improved patient safety in the prescribing step of care.

Evaluating the study environment for technology and information sources readiness revealed a startling finding: There is no patient safety framework for medications in primary care office practices. This led to the opportunity to conduct a comprehensive environmental survey to evaluate the safety needs of offices. From this, we have derived a "best practices" set of recommendations that we believe is a useful product.[8]

Finally, we considered the question of including the indication for a medication on a prescription blank. The finding that 78% of prescribers voluntarily will include the indication for a medication on a prescription by having that available as an easy to use option in electronic prescription-generation packages is meaningful to patient safety and may be more meaningful to the system of medication safety in the outpatient setting than some of the other questions we actually set out to answer.

Thus, what is appropriate evidence for patient safety? We need to consider that results of interviews, focus groups, and other forms of qualitative research can be confirmatory to decision making about safety. Learning the barriers encountered by prescribers through the interviews provided the evidence needed to make research-finding decisions about technology adaptation and adoption.

On the other hand, quantitative research, such as the use of the survey to assess the medication safety framework in the primary care offices, was exploratory and provided us with information for important new questions yet unanswered. The "good enough" evidence should be accepted for implementation as soon as such knowledge can be transferred for general consumption.

At the Second National Summit on Patient Safety Research: Updating the National Agenda, short-, intermediate-, and long-term questions were identified to help us address the evidentiary needs for improving patient safety long term.[9] These questions were offered:

Short Term

- What level of evidence is required?
- How should the effectiveness of safety improvement efforts be measured?
- How will we measure unintended consequences?
- Can we catalogue successful evidence-based interventions?
- How can we best get leadership and governance involved in promoting and prioritizing safety?
- What can we learn from other industries?

Medium Term

- What interventions increase safety? How should these interventions be evaluated?
- What effect does training have on safety?
- What technologies are effective in improving safety?
- What procedural redesigns are effective in improving safety?
- How can technologies, drugs, and procedures be designed and tested to improve safe use prior to general marketing?
- How is simulation useful in training and premarket testing?
- How do we know whether interventions are realistic and applicable in routine practice environments?
- How can we best foster education of both professionals and nonprofessionals (e.g., through formal education, continuing health education, in-service training)?
- What working conditions improve or detract from patient safety (e.g., how do staffing ratios, the mix of skills among staff, and work/rest cycles influence patient safety)?
- How can research on safety improvement be integrated into training promptly?

Long Term

- What are the organizational changes or characteristics that affect safety?
- How does trust among healthcare professionals and between professionals and patients influence the culture of safety?
- What cultural, organizational, and leadership factors promote safety improvement?
- What factors foster or hinder reporting?
- How does an organization create a nonpunitive environment for improvement?
- What is the effect of design and structure on safety?

Four major issues have arisen as a result of the work done since the first Summit on Patient Safety Research. These challenges will need to be addressed for progress to be expedited:

> *Issue 1—The Paradigm Challenge.* The first issue is the "landscape" of practices that might reduce error rates and patient harm is not clearly bounded. Many potential practices are clinical in nature, but many more are not. Changes in administrative procedures, the physical layout of an

operating suite, the working conditions for nursing staff, and numerous other common-sense improvements can contribute to patient safety improvements. In many cases, the most effective way to achieve safer care may be to re-engineer a system in which multiple changes to practices and the environment are made simultaneously. It also is not clear how to delineate the boundary between practices that improve patient safety (by reducing patient harm due to mistakes) and practices that improve quality of care (by ensuring that the best practices are used for a given clinical need). The UCSF-Stanford EPC evidence report *Making Health Care Safer: A Critical Analysis of Patient Safety Practices* established the following criteria for selecting which practices to evaluate[5, p.31]:

1. The practice can be applied in the hospital setting or at the interface between inpatient and outpatient settings and can be applied to a broad range of healthcare conditions or procedures.
2. Evidence for the safety practices includes at least one study with a level 3 or higher study design and a level 2 outcome measure. For practices not specifically related to a diagnostic or therapeutic intervention, a level 3 outcome measure is adequate.

The National Quality Forum's report *Safe Practices for Better Healthcare* also presented a set of practices with accompanying evidence and discussed how evidence of effectiveness could take many forms, including:

- Research studies showing a direct connection between improved clinical outcomes (e.g., reduced mortality or morbidity) and the practice

- Experiential data (including broad expert agreement, widespread opinion, or professional consensus) showing that the practice is "obviously beneficial" or self-evident (i.e., the practice absolutely constrains a potential problem or forces an improvement to occur, reduces reliance on memory, standardizes equipment or process steps, or promotes teamwork)

- Research findings or experiential data from nonhealthcare industries that should be substantially transferable to healthcare (e.g., repeat-back of verbal orders or standardizing abbreviations)[10, p.4]

Although both approaches are well thought out and are "correct," resource decisions will be very different depending on which of the two paradigms are followed. Leaders of healthcare organizations need further guidance about the pros and cons of the two approaches. Researchers and research funders also need clarification to integrate the two approaches.

Part of the clarification involves understanding different definitions of evidence, which is spelled out in issue 2.

Issue 2—Defining Evidence. The second issue is that for many patient safety practices it is not possible to evaluate performance using traditional scientific methods such as randomized clinical trials. The debate about the meaning of evidence is best exemplified in the two *JAMA* articles referenced previously; however, in the absence of the traditional scientific methods that have guided medical progress over the past half-century, what types of evidence should be added? What other types of evidence are there? How do we know when the practices from an "alternative evidence pathway" are good enough?

Practical research is key to identifying and implementing many patient safety improvements. Qualitative techniques (e.g., interview analysis, focus groups, case studies) are useful to describe processes and systems, essential knowledge for safety improvement. This form of investigation provides evidence in the practical world that may not meet the traditional standards of rigor associated with the science of measurement, but is legitimate and has a powerful influence on decision making. Combining qualitative with quantitative approaches using mixed methods may be helpful to determine the effectiveness of a change that is implemented to improve safety (measurement) while being able to understand why such a change was implemented successfully for future decision making (qualitative approaches).

The key issue is not deciding which approach is right and which is wrong but instead how to integrate the traditional evidence pathway that has served clinical medicine so well with a different platform that has led to success in other industries. We need to address this challenge to give guidance to healthcare organizations as they struggle with what safety practices to invest in.

Issue 3—Prioritizing Evidence. Healthcare organizations also need guidance in deciding between many practices that have acceptable evidence. Overall impact, cost and ease of implementation, patient preferences, and acceptability to medical staffs are all important considerations for the leadership of an organization. In medical practice, priorities are suggested by the use of practice guidelines or algorithms. For example, numerous studies prove efficacy in the treatment of hypertension, but translating multiple positive studies into the optimal treatment is done by the Joint National Committee on Prevention, Detection, Evaluation and Treatment. This committee, organized by the National Heart, Lung and Blood Institute, convenes scientific experts and acknowledged clinical leaders to develop a road map for treatment. For a field as complex as safety, nothing that could be construed as prescriptive would work, but there is a need to organize all of the positive evidence and help organizations prioritize.

Issue 4—Evidence About Effective Leadership and Organizational Change. How have other industries managed to make safety a top priority? In many aerospace and manufacturing businesses, zero defects is a goal pushed by the CEO, leadership team, and board of directors. Knowing that zero defects is a near unattainable goal, how did they commit the organization to this course? Because every industry has constrained resources, how did they decide between competing strategic priorities? Assuming that these industries did not have unassailable evidence from randomized controlled trials, how did leaders choose between interventions? Within health care, the improvements in safety in anesthesiology and in quality in selected healthcare organizations do not seem to be spreading sector wide. What can we learn about how change occurred in certain organizations that would be helpful to all leaders?

Evidence about how other sectors tackled safety issues and how certain organizations within health care have been successful is a gap in the current literature. It is critical that healthcare organizations learn from other industries and from success stories within health care—not just what practices were adopted, but also the ways in which leaders and organizations went about making decisions and transforming their organizations.

EVIDENCE IN SAFETY: AN ALTERNATIVE VIEW

The potential threat to patient safety resulting from errors in the medical research literature was discussed in Chapter 4. Two major factors contributed to errors in the research literature: improper experimental design and reporting and improper statistical analysis.[11] We now consider examples of these types of errors in the context of "evidence." That is, we examine specific errors that have occurred in the medical research literature in order to identify examples of "red flags" that a practitioner might use in determining whether a particular research report provides proper evidence of the safety and effectiveness of a medical treatment or a medical technology. Moreover, recognition of these types of errors might help practitioners avoid similar errors in their efforts to develop reliable measures of evidence related to patient safety.

Improper Experimental Design and Reporting

Issues related to improper experimental design and reporting may invalidate a research study. For example, in one case, a researcher categorized his subjects into a specific number of groups based on particular criteria; however, as the description of the research progressed, the number of groups changed, the definitions of the groups varied, and the number of subjects in each group changed. Furthermore, the definitions of the groups suggested that data for some subjects were included in more than one group. Of course, this led to double-counting problems that had a detrimental effect on the subsequent statistical analysis.

In another instance, an author claimed that his research was based on a specific number of subjects, whereas the reported demographic information included fewer subjects. Reported statistical test results also included fewer subjects, and the results for various tests included different numbers of subjects for each test.

In yet another case, data in scatter diagrams were inconsistent with the key to the diagram. Moreover, it was impossible for the conscientious reader to determine the types of subjects represented by the misidentified scatter points because the total number of data points (with or without the misidentified points) was inconsistent with the reported number of subjects in the study.

Although these types of experimental design and reporting errors can be frustrating to the reader, a more common type of error is much more frustrating. In many cases, the author does not report enough information about the experimental design to permit the reader to recognize the types of errors discussed previously. Moreover, inadequate reporting precludes replication of the study or expansion of the results by other investigators.

These types of problems are not a new phenomenon. For example, DerSimonian et al. examined all 67 clinical trials reported in *The New England Journal of Medicine, Lancet,* the *British Medical Journal,* and the *Journal of the American Medical Association* over a 6- to 12-month period from 1979–1980. Based on 11 important aspects of design and analysis, they concluded that only "56 percent were clearly reported, 10 percent were ambiguously mentioned, and 34% were not reported at all."[12, p.1332]

Improper Statistical Analysis

Major errors in statistical analysis have also invalidated research reports. The errors range from a mean follow-up time that is inconsistent with the raw data to less obvious (but perhaps more important) errors such as improper calculation of test statistics and the use of improper statistical tests.

In one case, the calculation of a t-statistic was based on the means of groups for which each group was treated as an individual observation in the computation of the test statistic and the degrees of freedom. Individual data values, not means, should have been used.

More importantly, the form of the t-test was incorrect. The test was conducted to determine whether there was a significant difference between preprocedure and postprocedure performance. Unfortunately, the form of the t-test that was used assumed that the samples were independent. This assumption is clearly violated in cases of preprocedure and postprocedure results for the same subjects. The correct form of the test in such a case is the t-test for paired observations.

In other instances, a fundamental assumption of the t-test was inconsistent with underlying population data. The t-test assumes that the underlying population data can be closely approximated by a normal distribution, a condition that may not be satisfied in a given research study.

Similarly, there have been instances in which a χ^2 test was used inappropriately. In one instance, the χ^2 test was used to test for "goodness of fit" between actual and predicted distributions. Unfortunately, a χ^2 test is not valid unless the expected frequency in each class is at least five, a requirement that, because of the small sample size in this case, was not satisfied.

Given the problems that arise from improper experimental design and reporting and improper statistical analysis, the caveat from Chapter 4 is worth repeating: Until appropriate changes are made in the healthcare education system, the onus is on practitioners to make explicit efforts to familiarize themselves with the decision sciences/medical informatics concepts necessary to evaluate the literature in order to ensure that they will not put patients at risk by basing treatment decisions on erroneous published material.

USING EVIDENCE TO AFFECT PATIENT SAFETY

Evidence is used in many different ways to affect patient safety. Evidence informs us across a spectrum of patient safety applications, e.g., from clinical decision making of health practitioners to formal system evaluation. Evidence in systems evaluation may be gathered through internal surveillance systems that include incident reporting, blame-free reporting, anonymous reporting, or a combination of these methods. Some systems encourage the reporting of near misses. These systems function well if timely feedback is provided and appreciation for reporting is expressed. It is also motivating (and necessary from a quality-improvement standpoint) to point out successes that result from this reporting to those who participate. There are also external surveillance systems, such as the JCAHO sentinel event reporting requirements and the use of surveillance systems in high-risk areas and during times of change.

Federally Recognized Patient Safety Organizations

In fall of 2008, the federal government finalized legislation that created federally certified Patient Safety Organizations (PSOs). A PSO is a public or private organization that collects, aggregates, and analyzes information related to quality and safety of the care provided in any healthcare setting. Voluntarily created under the Patient Safety and Quality Improvement Act of 2005, these organizations establish a framework for healthcare providers to report errors, "near misses," or other adverse patient safety events that cause harm to patients. The shared goal of all PSOs is to improve the safety and quality of healthcare delivery. As we move forward into the future, we will see the role of PSOs grow and be one of the contributing solutions to use of evidence to improve safety.

SUMMARY

The need to expand the definition of evidence to include qualitative, quantitative, and mixed-methods approaches to gathering evidence and accepting the validity and usefulness of these findings is clearly an important change in the advancement of patient safety that we must adopt. Implications to patient safety resultant from recognition and consideration of different evidence-based approaches are explored. Although we recognize the importance of having reliable, valid evidence, we also have grown to understand that contextual relevance of the use of evidence should guide us in finding the meaning and usefulness of evidence in all of its forms. We can gain value in the use of our research findings by using the different forms of evidence appropriately for the specific questions in patient safety that we need to address. There are many different ways that evidence is used to affect patient safety. Evidence to inform clinical decision making of health practitioners, informing system evaluation, and gathering evidence through internal and external surveillance systems are all important. The formation of federally certified PSOs is a recent step that will further our social mission of improving safety.

A CLOSING CASE

Read the following case and use the questions that follow to apply what you have learned in this chapter:

A student physical therapist is affiliating in a community hospital. The physical therapy department is taking the leadership role in an interdisciplinary evaluation of the hospital's fall-reduction program that was established in accordance with the Joint Commission 2009 National Patient Safety Goals.[13] Goal 9 is to reduce the risk of patient harm resulting from falls. Elements of performance for this goal include the following:

1. The hospital establishes a fall-reduction program.
2. The fall-reduction program includes an evaluation appropriate to the patient population, settings, and services provided.
3. The fall-reduction program includes interventions to reduce the patient's fall risk factors.
4. Staff receive education and training for the fall-reduction program.
5. The hospital educates the patient and, as needed, the family on the fall-reduction program and any individualized fall-reduction strategies.
6. The hospital evaluates the fall-reduction program to determine the effectiveness of the program.

The student's clinical instructor has invited her to participate. In preparation, the student begins to think about the types of evidence that might be used in evaluating the fall-reduction program.

1. If you were the student, what types of evidence might you expect the hospital to have gathered?
2. Choose one of the elements of performance and describe techniques (quantitative, qualitative, mixed methods) that might be used to gather evidence to support successful outcomes.
3. How can the hospital's use of evidence contribute to the improvement of patient safety by minimizing the harm from falls?

Discussion Questions to Launch Further Investigation

For further investigation, seek answers to these questions:

1. What kinds of patient safety questions would lend themselves to be answered by using qualitative methods of gathering information?
2. What are the potential benefits of using a mixed methods approach to answering patient safety research questions?
3. Why is there a need for external surveillance systems for patient safety?

REFERENCES

1. Leape LL, Berwick DM, Bates DW. What practices will most improve safety? Evidence-based medicine meets patient safety. *JAMA* 2002;288:501–507.
2. Shojania KG, Duncan BW, McDonald KM, Wachter RM. Safe but sound: patient safety meets evidence-based medicine. *JAMA* 2002;288:508–513.
3. Kuhn TS. *The Structure of Scientific Revolutions.* Chicago: University of Chicago Press; 1962.
4. Lohr KN. Comparative effectiveness and safety: emerging methods. *Med Care* 2007; 45(Suppl 2):S1–S172.
5. Shojania KG, Duncan BW, McDonald KM, Wachter RM, eds. *Making Health Care Safer: A Critical Analysis of Patient Safety Practices.* Rockville, MD: Agency for Healthcare Research and Quality; July 2001. AHRQ Publication No. 01-E058.
6. Galt KA, Rule A, Taylor W, et al. Impact of personal digital assistant devices on medication safety in primary care. In Henriksen K, Battles JB, Marks ES, Lewin DI, editors. *AHRQ Advances in Patient Safety: From Research to Implementation.* Vol. 3, Implementation issues. AHRQ Publication No. 05-0021-3. Rockville, MD: Agency for Healthcare Research and Quality; 2005;3:247–263.
7. Galt KA, Rich EC, Young WW, et al. Impact of hand-held technologies on medication errors in primary care. *Top Health Inform Manage* 2002;23:71–81.
8. Galt KA, Rule A, Clark BE, Bramble JD, Taylor W, Moores KG. Best practices in medication safety: areas for improvement in the primary care physician's office. In Henriksen K, Battles JB, Marks ES, Lewin DI, editors. *AHRQ Advances in Patient Safety: From Research to Implementation.* Vol 1. Research findings. AHRQ Publication No. 05-0021-01. Rockville, MD: Agency for Healthcare Research and Quality; 2005;1:101–129.
9. AHRQ Second National Summit on Patient Safety Research: Updating the Research Agenda and Moving Research to Practice. Crystal City, VA: November 7, 2003.
10. NQF Safe Practices Consensus Committee. *Safe Practices for Better Healthcare: A Consensus Report.* Washington, DC: The National Quality Forum; 2003.
11. Gleason JM. Decision sciences aspects of medical research. *Otolaryngol Head Neck Surg* 1988;98:101–103.
12. DerSimonian R, Charette LJ, McPeek B, Mosteller F. Reporting on methods in clinical trials. *N Engl J Med* 1982;306:1332–1337.
13. The Joint Commission. National Patient Safety Goals (Accreditation Program: Hospital). 2009. Available at: http://www.jointcommission.org/NR/rdonlyres/31666E86-E7F4-423E-9BE8-F05BD1CB0AA8/0/HAP_NPSG.pdf. Accessed March 31, 2009.

Taxonomy of Terms and the Source

Many working definitions for common terms used in the field of patient safety currently exist. This listing provides you with a summary of the most commonly recognized terms and definitions with cited references for the source of the definitions. In some cases, we have provided multiple definitions for the same term. This has been done so that you can appreciate the context of a definition that is used. For example, you may find it useful to know what the formal definition is for a term as recognized by the Joint Commission of Healthcare Organizations (JCAHO) as compared with the definition forwarded by the Institute of Medicine report *To Err Is Human*. Each definition has a citation for the source from which it was extracted. An additional resource that you may wish to continue to access periodically is the glossary of terms made available through the website http://toolkits.ehealthinitiative.org/glossary/.

Accident—(1) A series of events that involves damage to a defined system disrupting the ongoing or future output of the system.[1] (2) An unplanned, unexpected, and undesired event, usually with an adverse consequence.[2]

Active conditions/diagnoses—Information maintained in the patient record related to medical conditions or current diagnosed diseases.[3]

Active error—An error that occurs at the level of the front-line operator and whose effects are felt almost immediately.[1]

Active failure—(1) An error that is precipitated by the commission of errors and violations. These are difficult to anticipate and have an immediate adverse impact on safety by breaching, bypassing, or disabling existing defenses.[4]

(2) Errors and violations committed at the "sharp end" of the system—by pilots, air traffic controllers, police officers, insurance brokers, financial traders, ships crews, control room operators, maintenance personnel, and the like. Such unsafe acts are likely to have a direct impact on the safety of the system, and because of the immediacy of their adverse effects, these acts are termed active failures.[2]

Active medications—Medications a patient is currently taking. These include prescription medications, over-the-counter substances, nutritional supplements, natural products, and alternative medicines.[3]

Adoption of change—The process in which an individual embraces a new way to do something.[3]

Adverse drug event (ADE)—(1) An incident resulting from medical intervention related to a drug.[2] (2) Any incident in which the use of a medication (drug or biologic) at any dose, a medical device, or a special nutritional product (e.g., dietary supplement, infant formula, medical food) may have resulted in an adverse outcome in a patient.[4]

Adverse drug reaction (ADR)—An undesirable response associated with use of a drug that either compromises therapeutic efficacy, enhances toxicity, or both.[4]

Adverse event—(1) An injury resulting from a medical intervention.[1] (2) An injury that was caused by medical management and that results in measurable disability.[5] (3) An untoward, undesirable, usually unanticipated event, such as death of a patient, an employee, or a visitor in a healthcare organization. Incidents such as patient falls or improper administration of medications are also considered adverse events even if there is no permanent effect on the patient.[4] (4) An injury that was caused by medical mismanagement (rather than the underlying disease) and that prolonged the hospitalization, produced a disability at the time of discharge, or both.[6] (5) An event or omission arising during clinical care and causing physical or psychological injury to a patient.[7]

Adverse sentinel event—An unexpected occurrence involving death or serious physical or psychological injury or the risk thereof. Serious injury specifically includes the loss of limb or function.[8]

Allergy information—Information maintained in the patient chart related to allergies.[3]

Ambulatory surgical centers (ASCs)—These are medical facilities that specialize in elective same-day or outpatient surgical procedures. They do not offer emergency care.[3]

Automation failure (Safety Concern)—We should be able to react and respond to automation failures without compromising patients. Examples are as follows: equipment should be fail-safe, or alarms should signal; workaround plans should be available to recover from failures.[9]

Bad outcome—Failure to achieve a desired outcome of care.[1]

Benign errors—Events that cause no harm or lack an adverse outcome. This is also referred to as "precursor events" or "near misses."[2]

Birth defects, miscarriage, stillbirth, or birth with disease (Serious Adverse Reaction)—If exposure to a medical product before conception or during pregnancy is suspected of causing an adverse outcome in the child. (Examples include malformation in the child caused by the acne drug Accutane, generic name isotretinoin.)[1]

Blunt end—The blunt end of the system is the source of the resources and constraint that form the environment where practitioners work. The blunt end is also the source of demands for production that sharp end practitioners must meet.[2]

Board oversight—Management by overseeing the performance or operation of a person or group.[3]

Chart review—The retrospective review of the patient's complete written record by an expert for the purpose of a specific analysis. For patient safety, to identify possible adverse events by reviewing the physician and nursing progress notes and careful examination for certain indicators.[11]

Classification—A taxonomy that arranges or organizes like or related terms for easy retrieval.[11]

Classification system—The categorizing of errors into distinguishing levels based on their behavior, accountability, outcome, context, or process.[9]

Clinical data repository—A clinical database optimized for storage and retrieval for information on individual patients and used to support patient care and daily operations.[12]

Clinical records (medical records)—A chronological written account of a patient's examination and treatment that includes the patient's medical history and complaints, the physician's physical findings, the results of diagnostic tests and procedures, and medications and therapeutic procedures.[3]

Close call—See Near miss.

Cognitive science—An amalgamation of disciplines, including artificial intelligence, neuroscience, philosophy, and psychology. Within cognitive science, cognitive psychology is an umbrella discipline for those interested in cognitive activities such as perception, learning, memory, language, concept formation, problem solving, and thinking.[2]

Communication—Behaviors that increase risk to patients in operating theaters, including failure to inform team of patient's problem (e.g., surgeon fails to inform anesthetist of use of drug before blood pressure is seriously affected) and failure to discuss alternative procedures.[9]

Communication breakdown (related to treatment plan) (Safety Concern)—Discrepancies in communication of treatment plan between caregiver and patient or between two caregivers.[9]

Communications error (from aviation)—Missing or wrong information exchange or misinterpretation (e.g., misunderstood altitude clearance).[9]

Compliance regulations—Accurately following the federal or state regulations. A compliance program is a self-monitoring system of checks and balances to ensure that an organization consistently complies with applicable laws relating to its business activities.[3]

Complication—A detrimental patient condition that arises during the process of providing health care, regardless of the setting in which the care is provided. For instance, perforation, hemorrhage, bacteremia, and adverse reactions to medication (particularly in the elderly) are four complications of colonoscopy and its associated anesthesia and sedation. A complication may prolong an inpatient's length of stay or lead to other undesirable outcomes.[4]

Constraint and forcing strategies not available (Safety Concern)—There were no checkpoints or required steps that would force individuals to recognize the pending mistake. Some activities can be engineered so that it is impossible to make a mistake (e.g., it is impossible to attach an oxygen connector to the suction outlet because the connector is designed to fit only the O_2 outlet).[9]

Continuity of care record—A core data set to be sent to the next healthcare provider whenever a patient is referred, transferred, or otherwise uses different clinics, hospitals, or other providers. The continuity of care record will provide the necessary information to support continuity of care. The continuity of care record is a patient health summary standard and a way to create flexible documents that contain the most relevant and timely core clinical information about a patient and to send these electronically from one caregiver to another or to provide them directly to patients. It contains various sections—such as patient demographics, insurance information, diagnosis

and problem lists, medications, allergies, advance directives, and care plan—
that represent a "snap shot" of a patient's health that can be useful when
patients have their next clinical encounter. An ASTM International standard,
the standard, E 2369, Specification for Continuity of Care Record (CCR),
was developed by Subcommittee E31.28 on Electronic Health Records,
which is under the jurisdiction of Committee E31 on Healthcare Informatics (http://69.7.224.88/viewnews.aspx?newsID=772&s=E31; http://www.
centerforhit.org/x1105.xml).[3]

Critical incident—A human error or equipment failure that could have led (if
not discovered or corrected in time) or did lead to an undesirable outcome,
ranging from increased length of hospital stay to death.[2]

Critical incident technique—A set of procedures for collecting direct observations of human behavior in such a way as to facilitate their potential usefulness in solving practical problems and developing broad psychological
principles.[9]

Culture of safety—See Safety culture.

Data security—The process of protecting data from unauthorized access, use,
disclosure, destruction, modification, or disruption.[3]

Death (Serious Adverse Reaction)—If an adverse reaction to a medical product
is a suspected cause of a patient's death.[10]

Decision error (from aviation)—Decision that unnecessarily increases risk (e.g.,
unnecessary navigation through adverse weather).

Disability (Serious Adverse Reaction)—If the adverse reaction caused a significant or permanent change in a patient's body function, physical activities,
or quality of life (e.g., strokes or nervous system disorders brought on by
drug therapy).[10]

Dose omission—The failure to administer an ordered dose to a patient before the
next scheduled dose, if any. This excludes decisions by patients who refuse to
take a medication or a decision not to administer.[13]

Electronic health records—Extends the notion of an electronic medical record
to include the concept of cross-institutional data sharing. Thus, an electronic
health record contains data from a subset of each institution's electronic medical record (that is agreed on by the institution). An electronic health record
may also reside "entirely within one institution" and link the various affiliated
practice sites together. The electronic health record is generally patient focused

and spans episodes of care rather than a single encounter. An electronic health record can be present only if the participating sites all have an electronic medical record in place that is interoperable.[14]

Electronic medical record (EMR)—Generally defined as the set of databases (or repositories) that contains the health information for patients within a given institution or organization. Thus, an EMR contains the aggregated data sets gathered from a variety of clinical service delivery processes, including laboratory data, pharmacy data, patient registration data, radiology data, surgical procedures, clinic and inpatient notes, preventive care delivery, emergency department visits, billing information, and so on. Furthermore, an EMR contains clinical applications that can act on the data contained within this repository—for example, a clinical decision support system (CDSS), a computerized provider order entry system (CPOE), a controlled medical vocabulary, or a results-reporting system. In general terms, EMRs are clinician focused in that they enhance or augment the workflow of clinicians or administrators.[14]

Emergency medical personnel—Any persons that provide acute prehospital or out-of-hospital care. They are often linked with hospitals and usually either treat the malady or transport the patient to the next destination that will give urgent medical care.[3]

Emotional injury—Examples include elopement or "against medical advice" (also known as AMA), behavior health altercation between peers, wrongful confinement to a mental hospital, wrongful birth (birth after vasectomy, etc.), and fright, as well as fifth-degree sexual misconduct (touching or unacceptable sexual behavior, with no physical harm), and use of restraints.[15]

Environmental stressors (Safety Concern)—Workload, workspace, staffing, time pressures, noise, heat. Please identify specific factors contributing to the event.[9]

e-Prescribing—Electronic prescription (e-prescribing) writing is defined by the eHealth Initiative as "the use of computing devices to enter, modify, review, and output or communicate drug prescriptions." Although the term e-prescribing implies the use of a computer for any type of prescribing action, there is a wide range of e-prescribing activities with varying levels of sophistication:

Level 1—electronic reference handbook
Level 2—stand-alone prescription writer
Level 3—patient-specific prescription creation or refilling

Level 4—medication management (access to medication history, warnings, and alerts)

Level 5—connectivity to dispensing site

Level 6—integration with an electronic medical record

All levels of electronic prescription writing confer varying degrees of improvements in patient safety. Level 6, which is the most sophisticated, has been shown to confer the highest degree of patient safety and the largest return on the investment. Over the last 5 years, national interest in e-prescribing has increased as the Federal Government has enacted legislation including the Medicare Modernization Act, aimed at increasing the adoption of e-prescribing. Adapted from *Electronic Prescribing: Towards Maximum Value and Rapid Adoption*, eHealth Initiative, 2004.[3]

Error—(1) Failure of a planned action to be completed as intended or use of a wrong plan to achieve an aim; the accumulation of errors results in accidents.[1] (2) Failure to complete a planned action as intended, or the use of an incorrect plan of action to achieve a given aim.[7] (3) The failure of a planned action to be completed as intended or the use of a wrong plan to achieve an aim. Errors can include problems in practice, products, procedures, and systems.[5] *Note:* The JCAHO has taken a position on the definition of error. They recognize there are several definitions of error. "The terminology related to errors . . . in the health care world is far from fixed. There is a need to understand the error definitions being used in the context of patient safety initiatives in order to share a common understanding of problems, measures, and solutions."[9,16]

Error in judgment—Error related to flawed reasoning.[2]

Error, medical—The failure of a planned action to be completed as intended or the use of a wrong plan to achieve an aim.[17]

Error, medication—A medication error is any preventable event that may cause or lead to inappropriate medication use or patient harm while the medication is in the control of the healthcare professional, patient, or consumer. Such events may be related to professional practice, healthcare products, procedures, and systems, including prescribing; order communication; product labeling, packing, and nomenclature; compounding; dispensing; distribution; administration; education; monitoring; and use.[2]

Error of commission—An error that occurs as a result of an action taken. Examples include when a drug is administered at the wrong time, in the wrong dosage, or by using the wrong route; surgeries performed on the wrong side of the body; and transfusion errors involving blood cross-matched for another patient.[4]

Error of negligence—Error caused by inattention or lack of obligatory effort.[2]

Error of omission—An error that occurs as a result of an action not taken, for example, when a delay in performing an indicated cesarean section results in a fetal death, when a nurse omits a dose of a medication that should be administered, or when a patient suicide is associated with a lapse in carrying out frequent patient checks in a psychiatric unit. Errors of omission may or may not lead to adverse outcomes.[4]

Error Severity Codes[9]—

1. *Did not reach patient, potential injury*: Examples include a prescription bottle labeled correctly but nurse notices wrong pills in bottle, wrong medications loaded in Pyxis or med drawer, nursing station keeps all multidose medication vials in the same drawer or bin. The patient has to tell the laboratory technician not to take blood from a specific arm, no signs or notes on order or care plan, no sign in room.

2. *Reach patient: no injury or effect on patient*: Examples include missed antibiotics, double dose of pain medications, wrong laboratory tests done, wrong limb x-rayed, and diagnostic test done incorrectly.

3. *Emotional injury*: Examples include elopement or AMA, behavior health altercation between peers, wrongful confinement to a mental hospital, wrongful birth (birth after vasectomy, etc.), and fright, as well as fifth-degree sexual misconduct (touching or unacceptable sexual behavior, with no physical harm) and use of restraints.

4. *Minor temporary*: Minor patient injury or increased patient monitoring or change in treatment plan (with or without injury); length of stay increased by less than 1 day. Examples include an error in setting or monitoring heparin levels requiring increased number of laboratory tests, missed insulin dose requiring change in dosing for next administration, and/or increased glucose checks; bruising, abrasions, skin tear, complaints of pain, small number of nonfacial sutures; minor self-inflicted injury (scratches or cutting).

5. *Major temporary*: A temporary injury that exceeds minor temporary or increases length of stay one day or more. Examples include facial sutures, minor fractures, and a severe drug reaction.

6. *Minor permanent*: A permanent injury that does not compromise basic functions of daily living. Examples include a loss of finger, a loss of testicle

or ovary, removal of bowel because of circulatory compromise, a loss of teeth, second-degree sexual misconduct (forced sexual contact via threat of violence or weapon, forced sexual contact that causes injury, or sexual contact with someone younger than 16 years old), retained sponge/needle.

7. *Major permanent*: Permanent injury that affects basic functions of daily living. Examples include hip fracture, nerve damage from improper surgical positioning, missing limb, damage to sensory organ, first-degree sexual assault (forced sexual penetration via threat of violence or weapon, forced sexual penetration that causes injury, or sexual penetration of someone younger than 16 years old).

8. *Extreme*: Examples include brain damage, severe paralysis, and death.

Error, systems (or latent)—An error that is not the result of an individual's actions, but the predictable outcome of a series of actions and factors that comprise a diagnostic or treatment process.[5] The delayed consequences of a technical design, or organizational issues and decisions—also referred to as latent error.[15]

Event reporting—See Reportable occurrence.

Excessive handoffs (Safety Concern)—Information transfers and task handoffs become more error prone each time a hand-off occurs. Examples include change of shift issues, lunch breaks, ward secretaries performing order entry.[9]

Extreme—Examples include brain damage, severe paralysis, and death.[15]

Failure mode, effect, and criticality analysis—(1) The systematic assessment of a process or product that enables one to determine the location and mechanism of potential failures,[2] also abbreviated as FMECA. Another term used is failure mode and effect analysis (FMEA). (2) A systematic way of examining a design prospectively for possible ways in which failure can occur. It assumes that no matter how knowledgeable or careful people are, errors will occur in some situations and may even be likely to occur.[4]

Fault tree analysis—A systematic way of prospectively examining a design for possible ways in which failure can occur. The analysis considers the possible direct proximate causes that could lead to the event and seeks their origins. After this is accomplished, ways to avoid the proximate causes must be identified.[4]

Five rights of medication administration—Right patient, right drug, right dose, right time, and right route.[2]

Fixation error—The "persistent" failure to revise a diagnosis or plan in the face of readily available evidence that suggests a revision is necessary.[2]

Forcing functions—Something that prevents the behavior from continuing until the problem has been corrected.[18]

Genotype—Underlying mechanisms for patient safety problems, deeply root characteristics of healthcare systems. This includes latent failure in organizational structure or processes; safety culture and the blame process; organizational learning processes and barriers; production pressure; fundamental human limitations—performance-shaping factors; fatigue and sleep deprivation; stress; and human factors design in devices and systems.[15]

Genotype of an incident—(1) Patterns about how people, teams, and organizations coordinate activities, information, and problem solving to cope with the complexities of problems that arise. The surface characteristics [phenotype] of a near miss or adverse event are unique to a particular setting and people. Genotypical patterns reappear in many specific situations.[19] (2) The characteristic collection of factors that lead to the surface, phenotypical appearance of the event. Genotypes refer to patterns of contributing factors. They identify deeper characteristics that many superficially different phenotypes have in common.[2]

Harm—Death or temporary or permanent impairment of body function/structure requiring intervention.[13]

Hazard—Anything that can cause harm.[7]

Healthcare organization—Entity that provides, coordinates, and/or insures health and medical services for people.[1]

Health data (or information) exchange—The process of transmitting health information between systems is often referred to as clinical messaging or health data exchange.[14]

Health/electronic information interoperability—In health care, interoperability is the ability of different information technology and software applications to communicate; to exchange date accurately, effectively, and consistently; and to use the information that has been exchanged.[3]

Health information—Information in any form (oral, written, or otherwise) that relates to the past, present, or future physical or mental health of an individual. That information could be created or received by a healthcare provider, a health plan, a public health authority, an employer, a life insurer, a school, a university, or a healthcare clearinghouse. All health information is protected by state and federal confidentiality laws and by HIPAA privacy rules.[3]

Health information technology—Health informatics or medical informatics is the intersection of information science, medicine, and health care. It deals with the resources, devices, and methods required to optimize the acquisition, storage, retrieval, and use of information in health and biomedicine. Health informatics tools include not only computers but also clinical guidelines, formal medical terminologies, and information and communication systems.[3]

High-reliability organizations—Highly complex, technology-intensive organizations that operate, as far as humanly possible, to a failure-free standard.[2]

Hindsight bias—Finding out that an outcome has occurred increases its perceived likelihood. Judges are, however, unaware of the effect that outcome knowledge has on their perceptions. Thus, judges tend to believe that this relative inevitability was largely apparent in foresight, without the benefit of knowing what happened.[2]

Home health agencies—Home health agencies provide skilled care services in homes or alternative community settings. The Health Facilities and Emergency Medical Services Division is responsible for monitoring and evaluating the quality of healthcare services provided by certified home health providers and enforces Medicare and Medicaid standards in home health agencies.[3]

Hospice care—Facility or program providing care for the terminally ill. Hospice care involves a team-oriented approach that addresses the medical, physical, social, emotional, and spiritual needs of the patient. Hospice also provides support to the patient's family or caregiver as well. Hospice care is covered under Medicare Part A (Hospital Insurance).[3]

Hospitalization (Serious Adverse Reaction)—If a patient is admitted or has a prolonged hospital stay because of a serious adverse reaction (e.g., a serious allergic reaction to a product such as latex).[10]

Hospitals—Any institution duly licensed, certified, and operated as a hospital. "Hospital" does not include a convalescent facility, nursing home, or any institution or part thereof that is used principally as a convalescence facility, rest facility, nursing facility, or facility for the aged.[3]

Human factors—Study of the interrelationships between humans, the tools they use, and the environment in which they live and work.[1]

Iatrogenic—(1) (i) Resulting from the professional activities of physicians or, more broadly, from the activities of health professionals. Originally applied to disorders induced in the patient by autosuggestion based on a physician's examination, manner, or discussion, the term is currently applied to any undesirable condition in a patient occurring as a result of treatment by a physician (or other health professional), especially to infections acquired by the patient during the course of treatment. (ii) Pertaining to an illness or injury resulting from a procedure, therapy, or other element of care.[4]

(2) Any illness that resulted from a diagnostic procedure or from any form of therapy. In addition, we included harmful occurrences (i.e., injuries from a fall or decubitus ulcers) that were not a natural occurrence of the patient's disease; however, the term iatrogenic should not be construed to mean that there was any culpability on the part of the physician or hospital or that the illness was necessarily preventable.[2]

Improper dose—Resulting in overdosage, under dosage, or extra.[13]

Incident—Involved damage that is limited to parts of a unit, whether the failure disrupts the system or not.[2]

Incident reporting—A process used to document occurrences that are not consistent with routine hospital operation or patient care.[2]

Individual accidents—Ones in which a specific person or group is often both the agent and the victim of the accident. The consequences to the people concerned may be great, but their spread is limited.[2]

Individual errors—Those deriving primarily from deficiencies in the physician's own knowledge, skill, or attentiveness.[2]

Interoperability—When multiple information systems can seamlessly exchange health information messages, they are said to be interoperable. Electronic medical records are said to be interoperable if they are able to exchange (transmit and receive) data using standardized data transmission (coding and messaging) formats (standards).[14]

Interpersonal relations, conflict—Behaviors that increase risk to patients in operating theaters—overt hostility and frustration (e.g., patient deteriorates while the surgeon and anesthetist are in conflict over whether to terminate surgery after pneumothorax).[9]

Intervention—May include monitoring the patient's condition, change in therapy, or active medical or surgical treatment.[13]

Isolation—A means in industry to separate a process with high probability of failure from other processes to minimize the impact on the products being produced.[2]

Key stakeholders—A person or organization that has a legitimate interest in a project or entity.[3]

Lack of/limited access to information (Safety Concern)—No information or limited information available at the time. Our information systems, medical records, and decision support systems should give our employees the information they need when they need it. Examples include missing allergy information that could contribute to a medication error.[9]

Lack of training (Safety Concern)—Lack of training or inadequate training can leave our employees unprepared to perform. Staff members not oriented or not understanding the process.[9]

Lapses—Internal events that generally involve failures of memory.[20]

Latent condition—Preferred to latent error because it does not necessarily involve either error or failure.[20]

Latent error—Errors in the design, organization, training, or maintenance that lead to operator errors and whose effects typically lie dormant in the system for lengthy periods of time.[1]

Latent failure—(1) An error that is precipitated by a consequence of management and organizational processes and poses the greatest danger to complex systems. Latent failures cannot be foreseen, but if detected, they can be corrected before they contribute to mishaps.[4] (2) Delayed-action consequences of decisions taken in the upper echelons of the organization of the system. They relate to the design and construction of plant and equipment, the structure of the organization, planning and scheduling, training and selection, forecasting, budgeting, allocating resources, and the like. The adverse safety effects of these decisions may lie dormant for a very long time.[2]

Latent systems failures—Small, individually innocuous system faults that, if occurring in specific combination, can lead to catastrophic events.[9]

Leadership—Behaviors that increase risk to patients in operating theaters: failure to establish leadership for operating room team.[9]

Liability—One of the most significant words in the field of law. Liability means legal responsibility for one's acts or omissions. Failure of a person or entity to meet that responsibility leaves him, her, or it open to a lawsuit for any resulting damages.[21]

Life-threatening hazard (Serious Adverse Reaction)—If the patient was at risk of dying at the time of the adverse reaction or if it is suspected that continued use of a product would cause death (e.g., pacemaker breakdown or failure of an IV pump that could cause excessive drug dosing).[10]

Look-alike or sound-alike situation (Safety Concern)—Ambiguous labeling and nondistinct storage containers can lead to inappropriate use of medications or products. Examples are drug names that may look or sound similar, intravenous fluids that may be packaged alike, and reagent bottles that may be the same size and color.[9]

Major permanent—Permanent injury that affects basic functions of daily living. Examples include hip fracture, nerve damage from improper surgical positioning, missing limb, damage to sensory organ, and first-degree sexual assault (forced sexual penetration via threat of violence or weapon, forced sexual penetration that causes injury, or sexual penetration of someone younger than 16 years old).[15]

Major temporary—A temporary injury that exceeds minor temporary or increases length of stay one day or more. Examples include facial sutures, minor fractures, and severe drug reaction.[15]

Malpractice—(1) Negligent errors.[2] (2) Improper or unethical conduct or unreasonable lack of skill by a holder of a professional or official position, often applied to physicians, dentists, lawyers, and public officials to denote negligent or unskillful performance of duties when professional skills are obligatory. Malpractice is a cause of action for which damages are allowed.[4]

Medical error—(1) An adverse event or near miss that is preventable with the current state of medical knowledge.[5] (2) The failure of a planned action to be completed as intended or the use of a wrong plan to achieve an aim.[1]

Medical mistake—(1) A commission or an omission with potentially negative consequences for the patient that would have been judged wrong by skilled and knowledgeable peers at the time it occurred, independent of whether there were any negative consequences. This definition excludes the natural history of disease that does not respond to treatment and the foreseeable complications of a correctly performed procedure, as well as cases in which there is a reasonable disagreement over whether a mistake occurred.[2] (2) A commission or an omission with potentially negative consequences for the patient that would have been judged wrong by skilled and knowledgeable peers at the time it occurred, independent of whether there were any negative consequences.[3]

Medical technology—Techniques, drugs, equipment, and procedures used by healthcare professionals in delivering medical care to individuals and the systems within which such care is delivered.[1]

Medication error—A medication error is any preventable event that may cause or lead to inappropriate medication use or patient harm while the medication is in the control of the healthcare professional, patient, or consumer. Such events may be related to professional practice, healthcare products, procedures, and systems, including prescribing; order communication; product labeling, packing, and nomenclature; compounding; dispensing; distribution; administration; education; monitoring; and use.[2]

Medication Error Index[13]—

No error:

Category A—Circumstances or events that have the capacity to cause error.

Error, no harm*:

Category B—An error occurred but the medication did not reach the patient.
Category C—An error occurred that reached the patient but did not cause patient harm.
Category D—An error occurred that resulted in the need for increased patient monitoring but no patient harm.

Error, harm:

Category E—An error occurred that resulted in the need for treatment or intervention and caused temporary patient harm.
Category F—An error occurred that resulted in initial or prolonged hospitalization and caused temporary patient harm.
Category G—An error occurred that resulted in permanent patient harm.
Category H—An error occurred that resulted in a near-death event (e.g., cardiac arrest).

Error, death:

Category I—An error occurred that resulted in patient death.

Medication use information—Information related to the use of medication by a patient.[3]

Microsystem—Organizational unit built around the definition of repeatable core service competencies. Elements of a microsystem include (i) a core team of healthcare professionals, (ii) a defined population, (iii) carefully designed work processes, and (iv) an environment capable of linking information on all aspects

---

*Harm: death, or temporary or permanent impairment of body function/structure requiring intervention.

of work and patient or population outcomes to support ongoing evaluation of performance.[1]

Minor permanent—A permanent injury that does not compromise basic functions of daily living. Examples include a loss of finger, a loss of testicle or ovary, removal of bowel due to circulatory compromise, a loss of teeth, second-degree sexual misconduct (forced sexual contact via threat of violence or weapon, forced sexual contact that causes injury, or sexual contact with someone younger than 16 years old), and retained sponge/needle.[15]

Minor temporary—Minor patient injury or increased patient monitoring or change in treatment plan (with or without injury). Length of stay increased by less than one day. Examples include an error in setting or monitoring heparin levels requiring increased number of lab tests, missed insulin dose requiring change in dosing for next administration, and/or increased glucose checks; bruising, abrasions, skin tear, complaints of pain, small number of nonfacial sutures; and minor self-inflicted injury (scratches or cutting).[15]

Mispractice—Honest misjudgment.[2]

Mistake—The actions may conform exactly to the plan, but the plan is inadequate to achieve its intended outcome.[2]

Misuse—When an appropriate service has been selected but a preventable complication occurs and the patient does not receive the full potential benefit of the service.[2]

Monitoring error—Included contraindicated drugs resulting in a drug–drug interaction, drug–food/nutrient interaction, documented allergy, drug–disease interaction, or clinical reaction (blood glucose, prothrombin, blood pressure, etc.).[13]

Monitoring failure/vigilance failure—Those in which the essence is a failure to recognize or act on visible data requiring a response.[2]

Multiple entry (Safety Concern)—Multiple entry points for identical information can lead to conflicting or ambiguous data, or omissions. Examples include an allergy and height and weight information that can be entered into the patient record at multiple points in our system.[9]

Near miss—(1) A situation in which an event or omission, or a sequence of events or omissions, arising during clinical care fails to develop further, whether or not as the result of compensating action, thus preventing injury to a patient.[7] (2) An event or situation that could have resulted in an accident, injury, or illness, but did not, either by chance or through timely intervention.[4] This is also known as a close call or near hit.[9]

Needs intervention to avoid permanent damage (Serious Adverse Reaction)— If use of a medical product required medical or surgical treatment to prevent impairment (e.g., burns from radiation equipment or breakage of a screw supporting a bone fracture).[10]

Negligence—(1) Failure to use such care as a reasonably prudent and careful person would use under similar circumstances.[4] (2) Care that fell below the standard expected of physicians in their community.[6] (3) Failure to exercise the care toward others that a reasonable or prudent person would do in the circumstances or taking action that such a reasonable person would not. Negligence is accidental as distinguished from "intentional torts" (assault or trespass, for example) or from crimes, but a crime can also constitute negligence, such as reckless driving.[22]

Negligent injuries—By definition, in negligent injuries the standard of care and the procedures to prevent injury were well known, as well as the likelihood of serious injury if they are not followed.[2]

Nonstandard process (Safety Concern)—No procedure or process exists. When processes are improvised, there can be subtle differences between standard and nonstandard process that are missed in time-pressured situations. Examples include microwaving gel packs when not the manufacturer's recommended warming method, thus resulting in burns, taking shortcuts on procedures, and relying on folklore nursing techniques rather than following protocols.[9]

Normal accident—If interactive complexity and tight coupling-system characteristics inevitably will produce an accident, I believe we are justified in call it a "normal accident," or a "system accident." The odd term "normal accident" is meant to signal that, given the system characteristics, multiple and unexpected interactions of failures are inevitable. System accidents are uncommon, even rare; yet this is not all that reassuring if they can produce catastrophes.[23]

Omission—Failure to carry out some of the actions necessary to achieve a desired goal.[20]

Order transcription—Manually transcribed order leads to misinterpretation.[9]

Organizational accident—Comparatively rare, but often catastrophic, events that occur within complex modern technologies such as nuclear power plants, commercial aviation, the petrochemical industry, chemical process plants, marine and rail transport, banks, and stadiums. Organizational accidents have multiple causes involving many people operating at different levels of their respective companies.[2]

Overuse—When a healthcare service is provided under circumstances in which its potential for harm exceeds the benefit.[2]

Patient—An individual who receives care or services, or one who may be represented by an appropriately authorized person. For hospice providers, the patient and the patient's family is considered a single unit of care. Synonyms used by various healthcare fields include client, resident, customer, individual served, patient and family unit, consumer, and healthcare consumer.[23]

Patient permission—Expressed consent or authorization from the patient.[3]

Patient's privacy—For purposes of the HIPAA Privacy Rule, privacy means an individual's interest in limiting who has access to personal healthcare information. See also HIPAA Privacy Rule.[3]

Patient safety—(1) Freedom from accidental injury; ensuring patient safety involves the establishment of operational systems and processes that minimize the likelihood of errors and maximize the likelihood of intercepting them when they occur.[1] (2) Actions undertaken by individuals and organizations to protect healthcare recipients from being harmed by the effects of healthcare services.[2]

Perfectibility model—The perfectibility model is based on the notion that if a health practitioner were properly educated, trained, motivated, and ethical that he or she would not make mistakes that resulted in harm to patients; however, to err is human. The preoccupation on perfection and individual error has resulted in the creation of societal expectations that are unattainable and inhibits learning from errors and improving patient safety through system change.[24]

Personal health record—Refers to computer-based patient records intended primarily for use by consumers, which may or may not interface with providers' electronic records.[3]

Phenotype—(1) What happens, what people actually do or what they do wrong, and what you can observe. Phenotypes are specific to the local situation and context—the surface appearance of an incident.[2] (2) Safety problems; failures in specific health areas, that is, the superficial characteristics of the system as opposed to underlying mechanisms; prevalence and cause of medication errors by healthcare personnel in all settings; surgery or procedure on wrong part of body; errors in performance of hazardous activities (surgery, anesthesia, radiation therapy, etc.); misdiagnosis, selection of inappropriate treatment; and nosocomial infection (see also Genotype).[15]

Physical examinations findings—Information maintained in the patient chart relating to the condition of a person's health or physical fitness.[3]

Plan of care, progress, or consultation notes—Information maintained in the patient chart relating to management of health.[3]

Potential adverse drug event—An incident in which an error was made but no harm occurred (see also Near miss).[2]

Practice acts—A product, such as a statute, decree, or enactment, resulting from a decision by a legislative or judicial body.[3]

Preparation, planning, vigilance—Behaviors that increase risk to patients in operating theaters; failure to plan for contingencies in treatment plan and failure to monitor situation and other teams' activities (e.g., distracted anesthetist fails to note drop in blood pressure after monitor's power fails).[9]

Preventability—Implies that methods for averting a given injury are known and that an adverse event results from failures to apply that knowledge.[2]

Procedural error (from aviation)—Followed procedures with wrong execution (e.g., wrong entry into flight management computer).[9]

Proficiency error (from aviation)—Error caused by a lack of knowledge or skill (e.g., inability to program automation).[9]

Protocol/checklist inadequate (Safety Concern)—No checklist or incomplete checklist or checklist not used. Reference materials and checklists reduce reliance on memory. For example, the protocol might be not user friendly, incomplete, noncurrent, nonstandard terminology (metric vs. nonmetric, etc.), hard to follow, or complex.[9]

Proximal cause—(1) Not "true" cause but domains where the cause most likely exists.[28] (2) An act or omission that naturally and directly produces a consequence. It is the superficial or obvious cause for an occurrence. Treating only the "symptoms," or the proximate special cause, may lead to some short-term improvement, but will not prevent the variation from recurring.[4]

Quality of Care—(1) Degree to which health services for individuals and populations increase the likelihood of desired health outcomes and are consistent with current professional knowledge.[1] (2) The capacity of the elements of that care to achieve legitimate medical and nonmedical goals. Quality is, according to the Institute of Medicine, the degree to which health services for individuals and populations increase the likelihood of desired health outcomes and are consistent with current professional knowledge. Quality can be defined as a measure of the degree to which delivered health services meet established professional standards and judgments of value to consumers. Quality may also be seen as the degree to which actions taken or not taken maximize the probability of beneficial health outcomes and minimize risk and other untoward outcomes, given the existing state of medical science and art. Quality is frequently described as having three dimensions: quality of input resources, quality of the process of services delivery (the use of appropriate procedures for a given condition), and quality of outcome of service use (actual improvement in condition or reduction of harmful effects). Quality is how well the health plan or healthcare provider keeps its members or patients healthy or treats them when they are sick. Good quality health care means doing the right thing at the right time, in the right way, for the right person—and getting the best possible results. Quality programs are commonly called QA, TQM, QI, CQI—all referring to the process of monitoring quality in systematic ways.[3]

Radiologic information—Information that applies to anything procedurally, surgically, or therapeutically that involves radiology.[3]

Reach patient—no injury or effect on patient—Examples include missed antibiotics, double dose of pain medications, wrong laboratory tests done, wrong limb x-rayed, and diagnostic test done incorrectly.[15]

Recognition and cues not effective (Safety Concern)—Our systems should be designed so that our people can easily recognize when systems begin to fail or have failed. For example, it should be easy to recognize that a person with a pacemaker is about to receive an MRI, and it should be easy for staff to recognize and question abnormalities in a process or procedure.[9]

Regional Health Information Organization (RHIO)—A RHIO is an electronic network for exchanging patient health information among providers.[3]

Reliance on human checks (or rechecks) (Safety Concern)—Processes that rely on double-checking or triple-checking are prone to error.[9]

Reliance on memory (Safety Concern)—No tools or "memory aids" to assist in guiding individuals through the process of tools not used. (Human memory degrades as time goes by. Reliance on memory during multi-tasking is highly error prone.) Examples include not checking the medication administration record (MAR), verbal hand-offs versus written, not referring to an available protocol.[9]

Reliance on vigilance (Safety Concern)—Process relies on frequent or constant observation to ensure accuracy. For example, humans make poor monitors because they can be easily distracted. An IV pump is more reliable than a nurse in the ongoing monitoring of the rate of infusion; patients may fall when not supervised.[9]

Reportable occurrence—An event, situation, or process that contributes to or has the potential to contribute to a patient or visitor injury or degrade our ability to provide optimal patient care. Reportable occurrences can generally be divided into the following types based on severity: sentinel events, patient and visitor injuries (adverse events), nears misses, and safety concerns.[9]

Risk—The likelihood, high or low, that somebody or something will be harmed by a hazard, multiplied by the severity of the potential harm.[7]

Risk containment—Immediate actions taken to safeguard patients from a repetition of an unwanted occurrence. Actions may involve removing and sequestering drug stocks from pharmacy shelves and checking or replacing oxygen supplies or specific medical devices.[4]

Risk management—(1) In the context of hospital operations, the term "risk management" usually refers to self-protective activities meant to prevent real or potential threats of financial loss due to accident, injury, or medical malpractice.[2] (2) Clinical and administrative activities undertaken to identify, evaluate, and reduce the risk of injury to patients, staff, and visitors and the risk of loss to the organization itself.[4]

Root cause—A root cause is the most fundamental reason an event has occurred.[9]

Root cause analysis—A process for identifying the basic or causal factor or factors that underlie variation in performance, including the occurrence or possible occurrence of a sentinel event.[8]

Rule-based behavior—Familiar procedures applied to frequent decision making.[2]

Rural health clinics—A public or private hospital, clinic, or physician practice designated by the federal government as in compliance with the Rural Health Clinics Act (Public Law 95-210). The practice must be located in a medically underserved area or a health professions shortage area and use a physician assistant and/or nurse practitioner to deliver services. A rural health clinic must be licensed by the state and provide preventive services. These providers are usually qualified for special compensations, reimbursements, and exemptions.[3]

Safety—The degree to which the risk of an intervention (e.g., the use of a drug or a procedure) and the risk in the care environment are reduced for the patient and other persons, including healthcare practitioners.[23]

Safety concern—Protocols, procedures, products, or equipment that are problem prone or risk-generating processes that may degrade our ability to provide optimal patient care.[9]

Safety culture—Five attributes of a safety culture—these are the five high-level attributes of a "safety culture" that we strive to operationalize through the implementation of strong safety management systems.[9]

1. A culture in which *all* workers (including front-line staff, physicians, and administrators) accept responsibility or the safety of themselves, their coworkers, patients, and visitors.
2. Prioritizes safety above financial and operational goals.
3. Encourages and rewards the identification, communication, and resolution of safety issues.
4. Provides for organizational learning from accidents.
5. Provides appropriate resources, structure, and accountability to maintain effective safety systems.

Security and privacy barriers—A boundary or limit that presents maintenance of an individual's security and/or privacy.[3]

Sentinel event—An unexpected occurrence involving death or serious physical or psychological injury, or the risk thereof. Serious injury specifically includes loss of limb or function. The phrase "or the risk thereof" includes any process variation for which a recurrence would carry a significant chance of a serious adverse outcome. Such events are called "sentinel" because they signal the need for immediate investigation and response. This is a proprietary term developed by the JCAHO.[4]

Serious adverse reaction—A reaction that involves death, a life-threatening hazard; hospitalization; disability; birth defects, miscarriage, stillbirth, or birth with disease; or needs intervention to avoid permanent damage.[10]

Serious event—One that leads to or prolongs hospitalization, contributes to or causes death, or is associated with cancer or a congenital anomaly.[2]

Serious outcome—Death, a life-threatening condition, initial or prolonged hospitalization, disability, or congenital anomaly, or when intervention was required to prevent permanent impairment or damage.[2]

Sharp end—Where practitioners interact directly with the hazardous process in their roles as pilots, mechanics, air traffic controllers, and, in medicine, as nurses, physicians, technicians, pharmacists, and others.[2]

Sharp end of healthcare system—Practitioners at the sharp end actually interact with the hazardous process in their roles. In medicine, these practitioners are anesthesiologists, surgeons, nurses, and some technicians who are physically and temporally close to the patient.[25]

Skill-based behavior—Routine tasks requiring little or no conscious attention during execution.[2]

Slip—(1) Observable actions commonly associated with attentional or perceptional failures.[20] (2) An unintended error or execution of a correctly intended action.[2]

Standard—A minimum level of acceptable performance or results or excellent levels of performance or the range of acceptable performance or results. The American Society for Testing and Materials lists six types of standards: methods, specification, practice, terminology, guide, and classification.[1]

Standard classification—A systematic arrangement or division of materials, products, systems, or services into groups based on similar characteristics such as origin, composition, properties, or use.[1]

Standard guide—A series of options or instructions that do not recommend a specific course of action.[1]

Standard practice—A definitive procedure for performing one or more specific operations or functions that does not produce a test result.[1]

Standard specification—A precise statement of a set of requirements to be satisfied by a material, product, system, or service that also indicates the procedures for determining whether each of the requirements is satisfied.[1]

Standard terminology—A document comprised of terms, definitions of terms, descriptions of terms, explanations of symbols, abbreviations, or acronyms.[1]

Standard test method—A definitive procedure for the identification, measurement, and evaluation of one or more qualities, characteristics, or properties of a material, product, system, or service that produces a test result.[1]

Standardization—The process of establishing a technical standard among competing entities in a market, where this will bring benefits without hurting competition. It can also be viewed as a mechanism for optimizing economic use of scarce resources.[3]

System—(1) Set of interdependent elements interacting to achieve a common aim. These elements may be both human and nonhuman (equipment, technologies, etc.).[1] (2) A regularly interacting or interdependent group of items forming a unified whole.[5]

System complexity (Safety Concern)—Process with multiple steps and/or decision points. (A complex system requires excessive attention and can be tightly coupled.) For example, a surgical tray arrives missing a critical component or there is a delayed or erroneous laboratory result; if there are no contingencies for these types of events, they could be significant consequences.[9]

Systems approach—Using prompt, intensive investigation followed by multidisciplinary systems analysis to uncover both proximal and systemic causes of errors. It is based on the concept that although individuals make errors, characteristics of the systems within which they work can make errors more likely and also more difficult to detect and correct. Furthermore, it takes the position that although individuals must be responsible for the quality of their work, more errors will be eliminated by focusing on systems than on individuals. It substitutes inquiry for blame and focuses on circumstances rather than on character.[2]

Systems error—(1) An error that is not the result of an individual's actions but the predictable outcome of a series of actions and factors that comprise a diagnostic or treatment process.[5] (2) The delayed consequences of technical design or organizational issues and decisions. This is also referred to as a latent error.[2]

Telehealth—The use of telecommunications (i.e., wire, Internet, radio, optical or electromagnetic channels transmitting text, x-ray, images, records, voice, data, or video) to facilitate medical diagnosis, patient care, patient education, and/or medical learning. Professional services given to a patient through an interactive telecommunications system by a practitioner at a distant site. Many rural areas are finding uses for telehealth and telemedicine in providing oncology, home healthcare, emergency room services, radiology, and psychiatry among others. Telehealth services have been used between providers to provide supervision of one another and to provide evaluation of patients. Medicaid and Medicare provide some limited reimbursement for certain services provided to patients via telecommunication.[3]

Tort—French for "wrong," a civil wrong or wrongful act, whether intentional or accidental, from which injury occurs to another.[26]

Underlying cause—The system or process cause that allow for the proximate cause of an event to occur. Underlying causes may involve special-cause variation, common-cause variation, or both.[4]

Underuse—The failure to provide a healthcare service when it would have produced a favorable outcome for a patient.[2]

Unpreventable adverse event—An adverse event resulting from a complication that cannot be prevented given the current state of knowledge.[5]

Violation error (from aviation)—Conscious failure to adhere to procedures or regulation (e.g., performing a checklist from memory). [9]

Wrong time—Administration outside a predefined time interval from its scheduled administration time, as defined by each healthcare facility.[13]

REFERENCES

1. Kohn LT, Corrigan JM, Donaldson MS. *To Err Is Human: Building a Safer Health System.* Washington, DC: National Academy Press; 1999.
2. Zipperer LA, Cushman S, eds. *Lessons in Patient Safety.* Chicago: National Patient Safety Foundation. 2001. # 1-57947-188-9. Available at: http://store.patientsafetystore.org/. Accessed September 3, 2008.
3. eHealth Initiative Connecting Communities Toolkit. eHealth Initiative and Foundation. Available at: http://toolkits.ehealthinitiative.org/glossary. Accessed May 30, 2007.
4. Joint Commission on Accreditation of Healthcare Organizations. *Glossary of Terms.* Oakbrook Terrace, CA: Joint Commission on Accreditation of Healthcare Organizations; 2001.
5. Quality Interagency Coordination Task Force. *Doing What Counts for Patient Safety: Federal Actions to Reduce Medical Errors and Their Impact.* Washington, DC: Quality Interagency Coordination Task Force. Available at: http://www.quic.gov/report/toc.htm. Accessed November 4, 2002.
6. Brennan TA, Leape LL, Laird NM, et al. Incidence of adverse events and negligence in hospitalized patients: results of the Harvard Medical Practice Study I. *N Engl J Med* 1991;324:370–376.
7. NHS Choices. Homepage. Available at: http://www.nhs.uk. Accessed November 25, 2008.
8. Joint Commission on Accreditation of Healthcare Organizations. *Conducting a Root Cause Analysis in Response to a Sentinel Event.* Oakbrook Terrace, CA: Joint Commission on Accreditation of Healthcare Organizations; 1996.
9. National Patient Safety Foundation. National Patient Safety Foundation: Definitions List. Available at: http://www.npsf.org/rc/mp/definitions.php. Accessed November 25, 2008.
10. Henkel J. *Medwatch: FDA's "Heads Up" on Medical Product Safety.* Washington DC: Food and Drug Administration. Available at: http://www.fda.gov/fdac/features/1998/698_med.html. Accessed November 15, 2002.
11. Aspen P. *Patient Safety: Achieving a New Standard for Care.* Washington, DC: National Academies Press; 2004.
12. Rosenthal MM, Sutcliffe KM, eds. *Medical Error: What Do We Know, What Do We Do?* San Francisco: Jossey-Bass; 2002.
13. National Coordinating Council for Medication Error Reporting and Prevention (NCCMERP). *Taxonomy of Medication Errors.* Hague, Netherlands: National

Coordinating Council for Medication Error Reporting and Prevention (NCCMERP). Available at: http://www.nccmerp.org/pdf/taxo2001-07-31.pdf. Accessed September 3, 2008.

14. Agency for Healthcare Research and Quality (AHRQ). Available at: http://www. ahrq.gov/. Accessed November 25, 2008.

15. National Patient Safety Foundation. *Agenda for Research and Development in Patient Safety.* Chicago: National Patient Safety Foundation. Available at: http://npsf.org/ download/researchagenda.pdf. Accessed October 5, 2002.

16. Joint Commission on Accreditation of Healthcare Organizations. *Medication Use: A Systems Approach to Reducing Errors.* Oakbrook Terrace, IL: Joint Commission on Accreditation of Healthcare Organizations; 1998.

17. Institute of Medicine. Available at: http://www.iom.edu/. Accessed, November 25, 2008.

18. Reason JT. *Human Error.* Cambridge, UK: Cambridge University Press; 1990.

19. Woods DD. *Behind Human Error: Human Factors Research to Improve Patient Safety.* Washington, DC: American Psychological Association. Available at: http://www.apa. org/ppo/issues/shumfactors2.html. Accessed June 24, 2002.

20. Reason JT. *Managing the Risks of Organizational Accidents.* Aldershof, UK: Ashgate; 1997.

21. Law.com. Law Dictionary. Available at: http://dictionary.law.com/default2.asp?selected =1151&bold=liability||. Accessed December 2, 2008.

22. Joint Commission on Accreditation of Healthcare Organizations. *What Every Hospital Should Know About Sentinel Events.* Oakbrook Terrace, CA: Joint Commission on Accreditation of Healthcare Organizations; 2000.

23. Perrow C. *Normal Accidents: Living With High Risk Technologies.* Princeton, NJ: Princeton University Press; 1999.

24. Leape LL. Error in medicine. *JAMA* 1994;272:1851.

25. Cook RI, Woods DD, Miller C. *Tale of Two Stories: Contrasting Views of Patient Safety.* Chicago: National Patient Safety Foundation; 1998. Available at: http://www.npsf.org/ rc/tts/front.html. Accessed September 3, 2008.

26. Law.com. Law Dictionary. Available at: http://dictionary.law.com/default2.asp? selected=2137&bold=tort||. Accessed December 2, 2008.

Index